Fashion:

Concept

to

Catwalk

First published in France 2007 by
Groupe Eyrolles as *Studio et Produits*
61, bd Saint-Germain
75240 Paris Cedex 05
www.editions-eyrolles.com

English language edition first published in Great Britain 2008
by A&C Black Publishers
38 Soho Square
London W1D 3HB
www.acblack.com

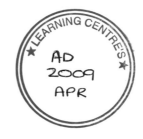

A CIP record for this book is available from the British Library

Ouvrage publie avec l'aide du Ministere francais charge de la
Culture – Centre National du Livre

Translation by Sasha Wardell
Cover design by Sutchinda Thompson

Printed and bound in China

studies in fashion

Fashion: concept to catwalk

Olivier Gerval

A & C Black   London

Contents

Preface

For more than 30 years fashion has been my life: not just its history and anecdotes but also the genius and high craftsmanship of French haute couture. To fully understand it in its truest sense, one must love it. Its vast universe, at times falsely criticised as artificial and futile is, in truth, simply a work of research, devotion and humility.

Which is most important? The garment, from conception to finish? The fashion designer's inspiration and the work of the studio? The fashion show and its team of models, make-up artists, and hairdressers who are supposed to present it in its best light? The space where it can be bought? Or the visual props which do their best to promote it in the shops?

From the dream to the drawings, or these 'little engravings' (as Mr. Dior called his sketches), to the choice of fabric, detail of the cloth and even to the manufacturing of this much-desired object, how much tension, anguish, application and labour, but also great pleasure goes into its execution! From the solitude of the designer to the hub of activity and skills of the production studio, or the arrival of the suppliers, this flowing ballet for a fleeting creation is illustrated in this first book of the 'Studies in Fashion' collection.

But, the garment itself, which is rejected from the outset by the fashion designer as he or she concentrates on their new collection, is bound to be out-of-fashion and quickly forgotten. Is it just a soulless piece of material to be thrown away? Saying that would be to ignore all the passion which comes with its creation and the care taken to give it identifiable and palpable qualities.

No! This book aims to place the garment firmly in context. Proving that it is enduring as well as being admired and cherished by the aficionados of style, elegance, art and beauty. The passing years have given it an unrivalled patina and a sense of mystery is linked to all the lives it touches. Likened to an exceptional wine vintage, with time it acquires a certain smoothness giving it its own identity. As you will have understood, vintage fashion is my passion giving me a favourable perspective on what is happening today in the fashion industry.

I defend the authenticity and charisma afforded to vintage fashion finding it quite wonderful. Imagine all the emotion when discovering Madame Grès' dress where the designer had inscribed 'not for sale', or the unparalleled structure of a Balenciaga coat having belonged to Mona Bismarck: the affinity of two beings on the quest for perfection.

Timelessness is, a dress from Schiaparelli's 'Circus' collection, a photo that Christian Dior dedicated to one of his French models, a piece of Bristol board with some words in blue ink by Cristóbal Balenciaga, some phrases from Chanel with her unforgettable voice, the youthful radiance of Jacques Fath ....And then, amongst all these unique and authentic wonders is the ultimate symbol of Parisian style and feminine elegance – the 'little black dress'. You will find several famous examples in the following pages. Omnipresent in the fashion scene for more than 80 years ever since Chanel's 'Ford', they are almost an obligatory 'rite of passage' for any aspiring designer which punctuate our memories now and then.

Balenciaga has used the 'little black dress' in each of his collections. Discreet, almost modest, yet unforgettable as a trademark or signature of his fashion shows.

One of the great merits of the 'Studies in Fashion' books is to pay homage to these talented craftspeople of taste, luxury and style. This book does just that by logically integrating all the necessary aspects and processes required in the production of a garment.

This is why I was delighted to accept Olivier Gerval's invitation to participate in his first book because the intrinsic nature of my profession is to share and impart knowledge.

Didier Ludot

Foreword

The 21st century sees a new chapter in the history of fashion. France loses its monopoly on this activity which had been inextricably linked with its history. The advent of new markets, delocalisation of manufacturing sites and the birth of a more demanding consumer defined new parameters for the designer.

The 1950s were synonymous with a particularly French expertise, that of *haute couture*. Its Pygmalions were designers such as Dior, Jacques Fath, Balmain to name but a few.

By the time the 'space race' was in full flight these big names had started to wane as already designers and street fashion had become symbiotic of which Pierre Cardin was the self-made ambassador.

The American dream had died in Vietnam, with the younger generation and the hippie movement strongly contesting consumerism; Antonioni's film *Blow-up*, Veruschka and Mary Quant coincided with the first oil crisis; design was no longer in fashion. Flower power epitomised the return to one's roots and the importance of the craft industry.

At the end of the 1970s, music dictated fashion. *Saturday Night Fever* prevailed over good taste. For designers such as Malcolm Maclaren and Vivienne Westwood, who together founded the Punk movement, the world was their oyster. It was also the start of Japanese fashion designers to come to the fore with people such as Kenzo, Issey Miyake, Rei Kawakubo (Comme des Garçons) and Yohji Yamamoto who collaborated with the film director Wim Wenders. They established a trend by introducing a concept into their collections. At the beginning of the 1980s a new start took place with the birth of the fashion designer.

The consumers' craze for designer-labels coupled with the media impact of fashion designers on the public, led financial groups to consider more closely the *prêt-a-porter* or 'ready-to-wear' sector of the fashion industry. LVMH (Louis Vuitton, Moet Hennessy), Richemont, PPR (Pinault-Printemps-Redoute) took over certain market sectors by creating artistic directors in order to personalise a company's image. As well as clothing, these extended into other consumer areas most notably accessories or cosmetics. The brand image and the personality of the artistic director had a notable effect on a garment. For example, Tom Ford was synonymous with the Gucci label in the 1990s, whereas Marc Jacobs with Louis Vuitton and Alber Elbaz with Lanvin illustrate this type of collaboration nowadays.

So many transformations necessitate a new approach towards the fashion industry, whilst specialist knowledge and a global understanding of the textile industry are fast becoming indispensable. The designer can no longer ignore the balance which exists between creativity, image control and commercialisation; it is the belief that fashion is a 'product' coupled with a continuing creative research which allows designers to be successful nowadays. It is also a necessary requirement to adopt a work ethic which is adapted to market demands.

The *Studies in Fashion* books originated from a desire to share my diverse professional experiences in France, the United

States as well as in Asia, notably Japan. This is done by echoing a schools' teaching programme which I perfected for secondary education. The aim of which is to give young designers a global vision of the fashion world in order to familiarise them with the professional sector.

The complete series aims to thoroughly and comprehensively present fashion and its related trades. Each book is independent of each other, with an analysis of techniques, knowledge and working methods from the great masters of the trade including an insight into their studios and ateliers. It describes all the skills and trades connected with our industry taking into account their transformations and relocations.

Fashion: Concept to Catwalk presents two types of creative areas. One of which is practised by the fashion designer and is simply termed 'products' and the other, the conceptual side, which belongs to the designer. Advice is given regarding the visual organisation of the 'material' at the research stage – mood boards, silhouettes, illustrations, finishing details etc., all of which assist the apprentice designer to present his or her work to its best advantage. The production stage in the atelier, ranging from the technical drawing to the making-up of the garment, must be perfectly mastered. This is thoroughly illustrated by means of an example which has been described in the previous chapters concerned with the concept of the idea. Eventually the product becomes a finished outfit, including accessories, as the book follows its journey culminating in its promotion and marketing.

Fashion: Concept to Catwalk is the result of many exchanges between professionals such as Didier Ludot, Lutz, Stéphane Marais, Odile Gilbert, Rebecca Leach, Stephan Schopferer, Martine Adrien, Antoine Kruk .... Like the other books in the series, it describes the knowledge and techniques belonging to the French heritage which have been so fittingly represented by Jeanne Lanvin, Sonia Rykiel, Christian Louboutin, Loulou de la Falaise and Louis Vuitton. We have at our disposal the creative starting points of these prestigious labels right through to their commercial strategies.

The label Lutz which has been chosen to present the fashion show clearly demonstrates this evolution. With an average size company such as this, it is just as important to satisfy its clientele as it is to respond to the demands of the boutiques. In our opinion this case history seemed more informative than that of a large company with the media impact which ensues.

If the *Studies in Fashion* books have been conceived primarily to appeal to young designers wishing to work for large brand names within the international textile industry then, hopefully, it will equally attract a larger audience who are curious to discover what goes on behind the scenes of this trade. Fully illustrated and constructed in the same vein as the fashion and design magazines, these books aim to appeal to all of those interested in fashion – a passion which is part of my daily life and which I fervently wish to share.

What we understand by the word 'products' are clothes which are normally destined for a wide audience known as *prêt-à-porter* or ready-to-wear (top-end of the market). However, the creation of such a line of commercial products does not, in the least, imply a lack of originality.

The word *prêt-à-porter* appeared in the 1960s with designers such as Pierre Cardin, Emmanuelle Kahn and Christiane Bailly and their desire to democratise 'couture' by making it accessible to the person in the street. Today, we observe the opposite of this phenomenon as collections actually adopt the influence of the street. This shows that if the product is commercialised it is inextricably linked to a certain historical and sociological context.

From the huge range of existing products, we have chosen to concentrate on women's *prêt-à-porter*. A certain number of them will be presented to the reader accompanied by detailed descriptions. We will also explain how to conduct preliminary research necessary for the development of coherent product lines, as well as how to define the theme of a collection.

Louise Brooks, Marlène Dietrich, Greta Garbo, Jackie Kennedy, Grace Kelly and Audrey Hepburn are all personalities from the past who, through their photographs, have contributed to the glamorisation of our dreams. They incarnate the fashion of their time and have defined past styles to posterity. The modern muses for designers now are actresses, rock stars and

Top models such as Nicole Kidman, Sarah Jessica Parker, Madonna, Beyoncé, Jennifer Lopez, Kate Moss, Naomi Campbell, Laetitia Casta without forgetting the veritable fashion phenomenon – Paris Hilton! This has the effect of making them seem more accessible.

With reference to these past icons, you will discover the private collection of Didier Ludot's vintage fashion – his 'little black dresses' being the glamorous items of a woman's wardrobe. Then, to introduce the world of the young designer to the reader, Lutz, ex-assistant to Martin Margiela, will explain his approach to clothing and the notion of the 'remake' – timeless clothing reinterpreted for contemporary trends.

The premise of a good collection is to find the right 'silhouette' – this is essential for a designer. We will show how to elaborate successful silhouettes which contain all the wealth and originality of a collection as well as clearly expressing a brand identity.

We will then demonstrate the construction phase of the collection by defining the colour ranges and harmonies relating to the seasons plus print and embroidery patterns.

Finally, we will show how all this work culminates in a collection plan and ultimately how it is made ready for merchandising and marketing.

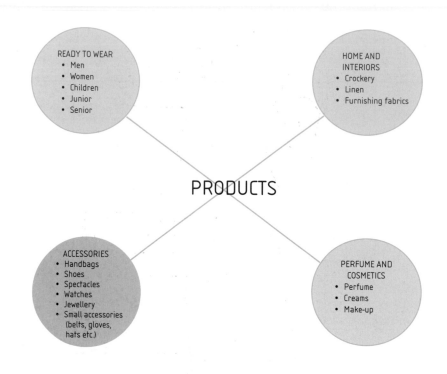

Sectors and industries

Fashion products are sold through boutiques, department stores (Harrods, Selfridges), large chain stores (H&M, Zara, Topshop), supermarkets as well as by mail order, through catalogues and e-commerce. They are distributed between sectors: clothing, or ready-to-wear, as well as accessories, perfumes and cosmetics, home and interiors.

Nowadays, the industry concerns itself with products which are directly linked to a policy of brand exploitation with larger conglomerates absorbing more and more specialised distributors. For example, the group LVMH uses Sephora to entice customers to a feast of cosmetics and perfumes with the help of attentive assistants who replace the erstwhile perfumers.

The designer has to remain alert to the consumers' ever-changing fashion trends. Too large a specialisation, for example, with print or jewellery, could result in a 'dead-end' if fashion reverted back to a minimalist trend as well as being detrimental to other products. It is infinitely better to be versatile and adopt a global view of fashion and its diverse sectors.

Manufacturing costs are too high in developed countries for the majority of products in comparison to emerging countries such as China and India where wages are low and the industries are heavily subsidised. This delocalisation coupled with global trading requires new strengths. Therefore, above and beyond possessing a sound knowledge of the product, the designer must also have a good understanding of geopolitics, international law, economics and sociology. It is also an advantage to be multilingual in order to converse with foreign production sites and representatives.

The textile industry makes products for men, women and children: from babies, infants, juniors, teenagers to even the family pet. As it is impossible to include all of this in one book, we have chosen to concentrate on womenswear (ready-to-wear).

This branch of *prêt-à-porter* is divided into several sectors: knitwear (jerseys and sweaters), sportswear, casual wear and underwear. It is worth noting that, within these sectors, there are also products which are under licence: for example, a specialist jersey manufacturer can make an assurance to produce and distribute a product for a brand which in turn will receive royalties.

Women's *prêt-à-porter* can also integrate more elitist sectors. In fact, if Paris manages to maintain its privileged position as the capital of the fashion world, it is thanks to its specialist knowledge of *haute couture*. This is understood by many large groups so, to stem the competition from emerging countries, they will buy up specialist artisans' studios which are on the point of disappearing – a particular example of this is the buy-out of the embroiderer François Lesage by Chanel in 2002 thus saving it from near bankruptcy.

An essential principle: lengths

In the history of costume and fashion the length of women's clothing varied depending on the economic and social context. This in turn became a determining factor of fashion.

For example, at the beginning of the 20th century, women wore long hemlines. Then, with the advent of the First World War which was a decisive period in the emancipation of women, they wore more practical clothing as they were obliged to work in factories and fields whilst the men went to the Front. In the 1920s this trend was ratified by the introduction of knee-length fashion illustrated by Chanel's 'tomboy' look.

Punctuated by the 1929 Wall Street crash and the ensuing Depression of the 1930s, a more austere fashion emerged which saw women returning to reassuring traditional values and longer hemlines again. The shortage of material in the 1940s resulted in a return to shorter fashions for women with the provocative style of the jazz swingers' long jackets and zoot suits. After the Second World War, Paris became, once more, the capital of elegance with the emergence of couturiers such as Jacques Fath, Hubert de Givenchy and Christian Dior whose New Look collection in 1947 spawned the calf-length fashion.

The 'space-race' of the 1960s inspired futuristic visionaries: fashions became radically shorter with the geometric forms of Courrèges, Pierre Cardin and Paco Rabanne. In the 1970s they lengthened again with *djellabas* and the peasant skirts adopted by the hippie movement, only to shorten once again in the 1980s with tailored suits designed for the career woman.

From the 1990s onwards, designers became interested in the notion of 'concept' (see Chapter 3). In an effort to create a strong personal identity, each one imposes their own length and style. Today, in an attempt to impress both the media and public alike, they aim to be the 'best of the season' with the concept being more important than the length. Trends define the 'indispensables' such as the trench coat and the safari jacket which each designer includes in his or her own style. The designer is then free to modify the shape and length within the body of the same collection. We advise apprentice designers to concentrate on one or two shapes maximum which will in turn naturally determine the lengths of their collections.

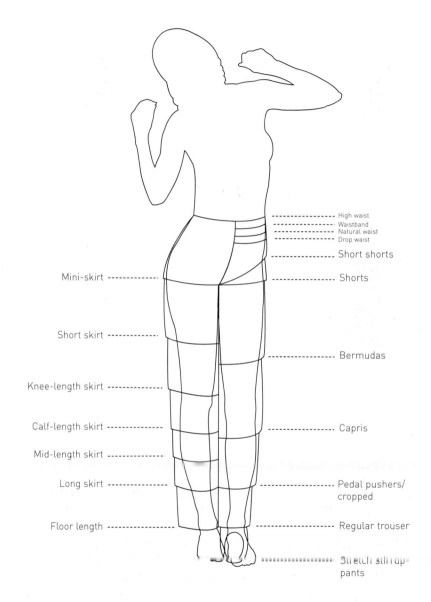

High waist
Waistband
Natural waist
Drop waist
Short shorts
Shorts
Mini-skirt
Bermudas
Short skirt
Knee-length skirt
Calf-length skirt
Capris
Mid-length skirt
Long skirt
Pedal pushers/ cropped
Floor length
Regular trouser
Stretch stirrup pants

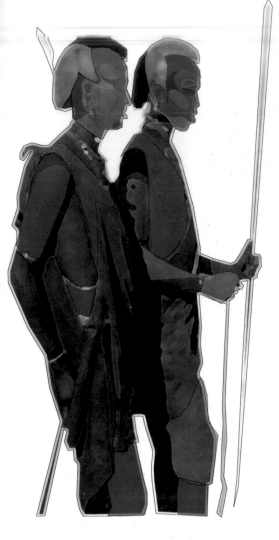

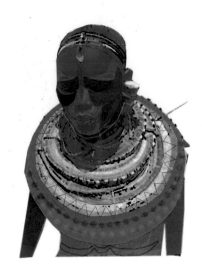

follow trends for their clientele, whereas others communicate to an already initiated following by means of a code. In this case, it is very important that the designer becomes a visionary who is able to produce an element of surprise and originality.

Women have always been a major source of inspiration for designers with many drawing on the feeling of adoration that women evoke. This then becomes their muse and, in turn, a theme. Contemporary fashion icons are inextricably linked to the impact of an image which bears a symbiotic collaboration between the designer, the woman and eventually the photographer who captures it all on film.

The muse

The muse can embody a style and remains a continual source of inspiration for the designer. Each season's collection is made up of different themes inspired by, or for, the muse. A good example of this is Thierry Mugler with Dauphine de Jerphanion – the style never varied whether she was represented as a Hollywood 'vamp' or was wearing motor biker's leathers. In this case, it is often difficult to dissociate the label's image from the muse's style. Although special relationships exist nowadays between a designer and a particular model, exclusivity is less frequent. The following associations are perhaps amongst some of the most famous: Jacques Fath and Bettina Graziani, Hubert de Givenchy and Audrey Hepburn, Mary Quant and Twiggy, Yves Saint Laurent and Loulou de la Falaise or Catherine Deneuve, Karl Lagerfeld and Inès de la Fressange for Chanel, Azzedine Alaïa and Naomi Campbell, Pierre Cardin and Hiroko Matsumoto ....

The subject of a collection is known as the 'theme'. And it is this which determines the shapes, colours and materials used. A collection can also have a principal theme which is developed through a series of sub-themes (see Chapter 3, pp. 86-9). The artistic director decides on the theme in consultation with the design team. It is here where the ideas are debated in a language particular to the fashion world; its technical vocabulary, codes and references must be mastered by the

designer so that he or she can communicate it to the rest of the team.

Thorough research is necessary to define a theme. This is done by looking at a number of sources including historical, ethnological, sociological as well as art and the natural world not forgetting the archives of the fashion house with whom the designer is working.

The designer who, in fact, is the trendsetter, must also be aware of what is happening in the arts, fashion, music and cinema, architecture, design, important current affairs and new technologies. In order to increase his or her inspiration, regular visits to museums, exhibitions and art galleries are indispensable.

Certain labels choose themes which

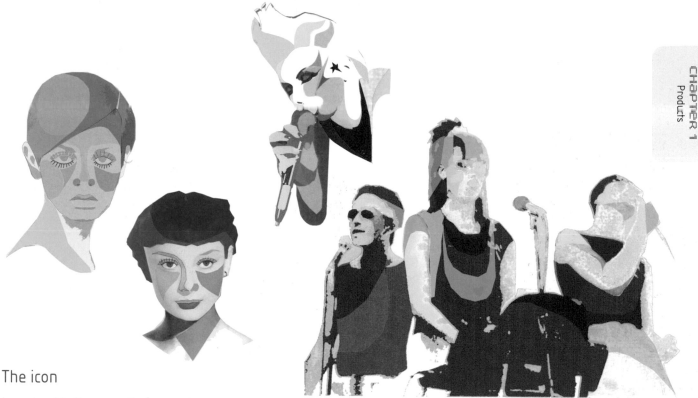

The icon

In contrast to the muse, the icon evokes a collective dream or idea. Her charisma is often more famous than the label she promotes. She is an ambassador for the fashion world and doesn't identify with any one designer even if she has a preference for one or another. She corresponds more to a style, or an era, and will lend her name to a product which has been specially made for her. For example, the Kelly handbag with Hermès and the Lady Di handbag with Dior.

Nowadays, icons such as Louise Brooks, Marlène Dietrich, Grace Kelly, Veruschka and Jackie Kennedy-Onassis illustrate the classical theme associated with their own 'couture' style.

Designers and celebrities

In the 1990s, top models such as Kate Moss or Naomi Campbell and actresses and singers such as Madonna, Beyoncé, Jennifer Lopez, Paris Hilton, to name but a few, as well as women in general, became great sources of inspiration as diverse as there are different types of women. Madonna's sexy stage bodices and exaggerated corsets by Jean Paul Gaultier became a strong image of this particular designer's collection. However, this approach linked to the media sometimes projects a simplified vision of fashion which can develop unnervingly quickly and at times is difficult to follow.

Collaborations with artists

Some themes originate from famous artistic collaborations such as Paul Poiret and Raoul Dufy, Coco Chanel and Sonia Delaunay, Yves Saint Laurent and Piet Mondrian and more recently Marc Jacobs with Louis Vuitton and Takashi Murakami where the artists' paintings are used as the theme for a line of bags.

Ethnic sources

These are also rich sources of inspiration. For example, John Galliano used the Masaï for one of his collections and Jean Paul Gaultier fascinated us with his theme of African masks. Oriental influence, in particular Japanese, was an important theme at the beginning of the last century not only for fashion but for art in general.

Classic items and new looks

The garment itself can be a theme with huge classics being reinvented – the trench coat being a good example. Work clothes such as overalls and military uniforms are often used as inspiration for shape, fabrics and details, e.g. safari and reefer jackets, sailor sweaters etc. Here the reference point is historical as well as ethnological where the past and the present meet.

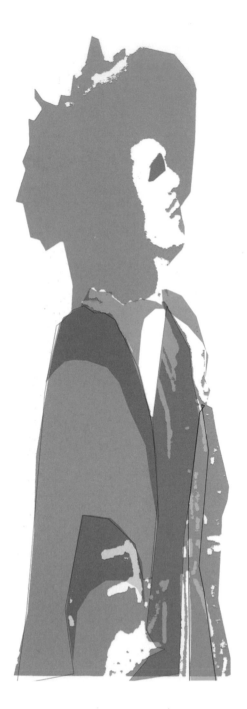

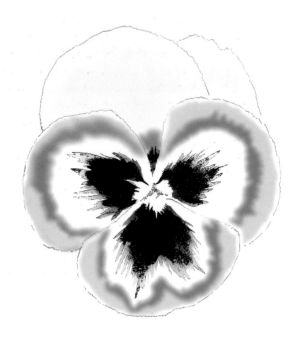

History itself has a rich variety of sources which can be used as research material. By offering common cultural references, which are always interesting to work with for a collection, it is omnipresent, from being studied at school, as well as interpreted through cinema, literature and the fine arts. Nothing escapes history not even our personal or collective memories. Places are impregnated by their history and we, in turn, belong to them.

Fashion itself has its own history – that which we perceive to be 'out of fashion'.

For the designer, the first point of interest is to build up his, or her, own historical reference bank and immerse oneself in a fashion culture thus acquiring a better understanding of clothing and its evolution.

Historical research is done by visiting museums and libraries. It is very important to find the source of the information rather than reinterpreting work which has itself been recuperated and would therefore lack substance and integrity. Through historical document-ation you will learn how to discriminate and interpret the facts themselves.

Interpretations

The further back in history, the more fictional and mythical the collective imagination becomes. There seems to be a somewhat distorted perception of past events which differ continually. We only have to look at historical films to convince ourselves of this as interpretation of the same subject varies from one generation to another.

Moreover, historical periods, or interpretations thereof, intermingle: for example, in the 19th century, the historical novel influenced fashion and even the habits of women of a particular era. Therefore the designer will need to keep in mind that history is constantly being rewritten and that he, or she, must draw on solid references to give the designs a true originality. A particularly good example of a designer who respects these factors is evident in the work of Yohji Yamamoto. He draws on tradesmen's clothing from the last century using professionals such as carpenters, cobblers and millers.

Updating an historical theme

In the fashion world research into the past can be very interesting when connected to the present. A good iconographic selection must be able to be updated. Good examples of this are the fitted coat and military uniforms which are regularly revisited by designers.

The difficulty is not to fall into the trap of creating theatrical costumes. Nevertheless, some artistic directors opt for this genre of clothing as with John Galliano for Dior whose themes have been Egyptian, Victorian and Marie Antoinette successively. However, it is worth noting that these fashion shows are aimed more at the promotion of a particular label than at 'high street' clothing. The young designer must bear in mind that to ignore business imperatives would be commercial suicide.

Sources of inspiration need to be used subtly, with just a hint of their origins apparent, and adapted to a current lifestyle. One can always use a cliché if it is in good taste and humour. An example of this being Jean Paul Gaultier who established his identity by reinventing sailors and market traders' clothing etc.

Our example

Research of historical themes allows the designer to imagine the outline, cut, finish and details borrowed from the past and reinterpret them with quality and originality.

The prototype we have chosen to develop throughout this book refers to the historical references of the peplum and gladiatorial armour. The contrast between femininity and virility illustrated by these historical costumes seemed to correspond perfectly to our current era. The draped dresses designed by Phoebe Philo for the Chloe summer collection of 2005 bear witness to this.

We have used the pansy flower as inspiration for patterns and motifs. The reason being that, associated with historical elements, the flower emphasises the fragile nature of this fashion.

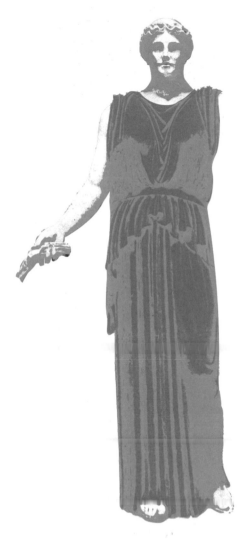

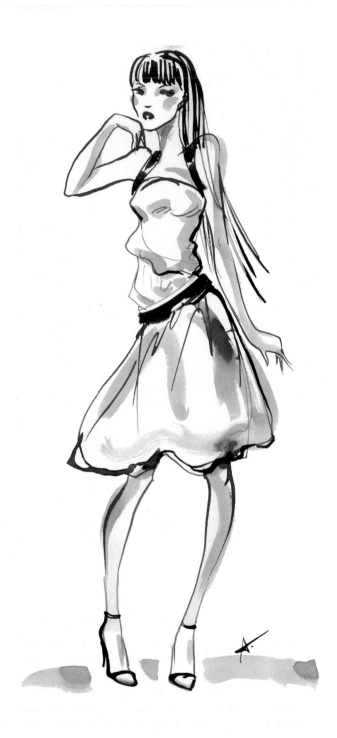

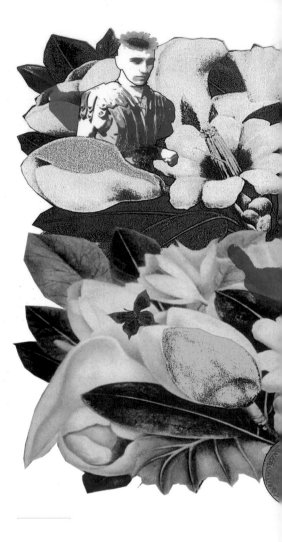

The designer will use the visuals found during his or her research to compose the storyboards – this will determine the collection's direction. Normally, one is made for the theme, one for the fabrics and one for the colour ways. They play an important part of the young designers' personal file or book (see Chapter 4 pp. 116-19) as these

COLOUR
PALETTE

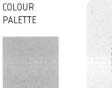

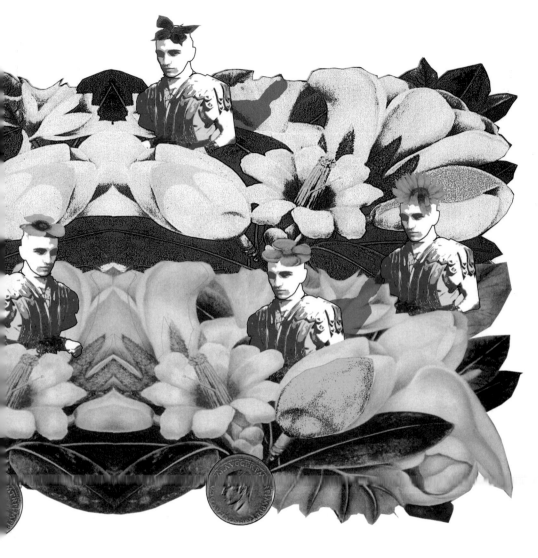

PANTONE® REFERENCES
PANTONE® PINK LAVENDER - 04-3207 TPX
PANTONE® PALE OLIVE GREEN - 15-0522 TPX
PANTONE® TAN - 16-1334 TPX
PANTONE® NAUTICAL BLUE - 19-4050 TPX
PANTONE® ELEPHANT SKIN - 17-0205 TPX
PANTONE® JET BLACK - 19-0303 TPX

assist with the coherence and possible directions of the project. In the studio, they will eventually be presented as boards so that the entire team can go forward in the same direction.

Storyboards illustrate the chosen theme in a balanced composition incorporating colour ways, fabric textures and suggestions of shape. They must also show an immediate understanding of the theme.

In the above example the gladiator's armour, with its image of virility, disappear in an abundance of flowers which instantly evoking femininity. The mix of pastel and sombre colours contribute to the paradoxical aspect of the composition whilst the flower textures inspire the use of fine fabrics such as silk and dupion.

The illustration on the left balances the page with reference to the colour chart on the right; all of which suggest a 'look' corresponding to a feeling or atmosphere (see Chapter 6, p. 173).

Didier Ludot's definition

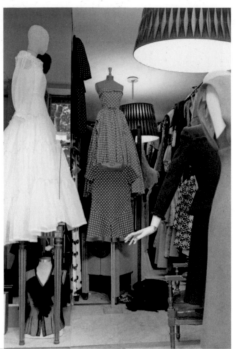

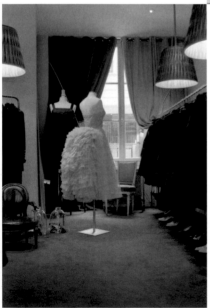

Vintage fashion is an elitist idea. The word itself, which is borrowed from the English winemakers' vocabulary, implies a 'great vintage'. Applied to the fashion world it likens a garment to this metaphor suggesting that it is a rare and authentic piece which represents the style of a particular couturier or era.

Yves Saint Laurent launched this trend with his 'war' collection in 1970-71. The retro look entered the couture world and Didier Ludot created a new metier: vintage fashion. However, being 'antique' is not an essential prerequisite – provided they are signed, the range can be very broad. Madeleine Vionnet's 'riding dress' and John Galliano's 'tramp' collection for Dior are good examples of this trend, however, 'secondhand' clothes are not included.

Vintage fashion is synonymous with quality in every sense by using only the very best fabrics which evoke luxury. It is a direct reflection of the unequalled knowledge of the French craftsmen and women which the suppliers to the couture industry strongly defend so that it does not disappear.

It is very much linked to Paris and France's heritage of *haute couture*.

A precarious resurgence of the latter has played an important part in a growing general interest in its history and never have retrospective fashion exhibitions been so vibrant.

One of the byproducts of teaching vintage fashion to the new breed of young designers means that the once-forgotten famous couturiers and fashion houses such as Martial and

THE VINTAGE FASHION BOUTIQUE BY DIDIER LUDOT AT THE PALAIS-ROYAL, MONTPENSIER GALLERY.
HERE ONE FEELS THE ATMOSPHERE OF THE BIG FASHION HOUSES WHERE THE CLOTHES ARE PRESENTED.

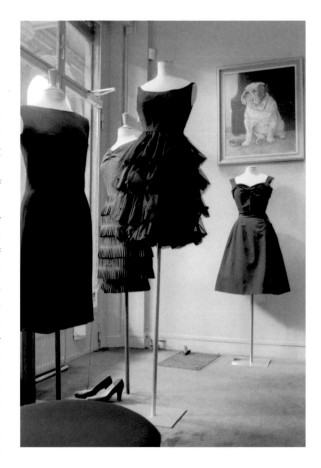

Armand, Louise Boulanger, Augusta Bernard, Agnès Drecoll, Maggy Rouff, Jacques Griffe, Jean Dessès, Marc Vaughan etc. are experiencing a revival, which in turn ensures the continuation of this trade.

If rarity is also one of the major factors of vintage fashion, it is because it requires, not only a collection of knowledge and patience, but also a desire and longing. The woman who has found the dress of her dreams becomes very attached to it, considering it to be a valuable asset which deserves preservation. Vintage clothing allows her to be her own stylist and, by discovering the playful spirit of the fashion world, she will be able to dress it up with accessories from her own wardrobe. Those most passionate about this will be able to build up their own 'museum' collection of vintage clothing breathing life into them again by wearing them.

The interest in vintage fashion has for a long time gone further than the fashion world and its aficionados. It is not simply the designers and fashion houses who seem determined to revive their archives, nor even the museums who wish to strengthen their collections, but it is more a sign of nostalgia for a quality of life considered lost by the younger generation. Vintage fashion is reassuring and comforting. A lasting and timeless addition to any woman's wardrobe which reinforces safe values and allows its owner to affirm her personality and originality due to its rarity factor.

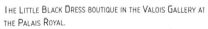
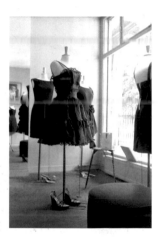

The Little Black Dress boutique in the Valois Gallery at the Palais Royal.
A setting which evokes a nightclub atmosphere where a ballerina might frequent.

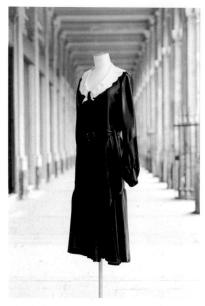

1927

CHANEL. 1927. SILK-SATIN DRESS INSPIRED BY CHAMBERMAIDS AND SCHOOLGIRLS UNIFORM. CORNELY-EMBROIDERED COLLAR MOUNTED ON ORGANDY. BAKELITE BUCKLED BELT. SAILOR DETAIL ON THE FRONT. FULL SLEEVES WITH STITCHED SEAMS ON THE ELBOW. GATHERED CUFFS. FLOUNCED.

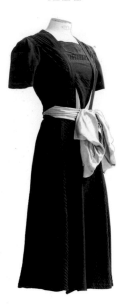

1936

AGNÈS DRECOLL. 1936. BLACK CRÊPE DRESS WITH SMOCKED YOKE. SHORT PUFF SLEEVES. ABSINTHE-COLOURED SILK-SATIN BELT WITH BOW.

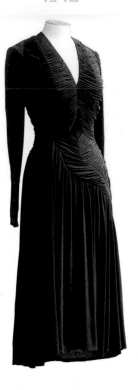

1942

MARCELLE ALIX (MADAME GRÈS). 1942. DRAPED JERSEY DRESS. ASYMMETRIC BACK AND FRONT.

The little black dress is the epitome of Parisian style. It is also a combination of contrasts: originating from widows and maids, it has become the symbol of the respectable woman who wants to seduce – a fantasy shared between men and women alike. In 1999, Didier Ludot* dedicated a boutique to it and every season since has created a collection of thirteen exclusive designs with the collaboration of the designer Felix Farrington.

Wearing a little black dress the woman experiences the playful spirit of fashion: to be seen, to deceive and to confuse the issue! In 1926 Chanel made it the symbol of Parisian chic by incorporating modern elegance with the tomboy look. Slim with short hair and wearing a knee-length dress with a pearl necklace are redolent of Paul Poiret's Sheherazade.

His 'Ford' dress is black and severe, similar to the cars of the famous puritan car manufacturer, but it is worth a small fortune and is only accessible to a rich and elegant elite.

The little black dress has however come onto the scene and has showed no sign of leaving. The 1930s saw it softened and lengthened, cut on the bias, accentuated by a white lining making it as romantic as those who wear it. Parisian *haute couture* was at the peak of its fame.

With the exception of Balenciaga whose fashion house opened in 1937, it was an exclusive privilege reserved for the following designers with their own particular characteristics : Vionnet – the bias, Chanel – style, Marcelle Alix (Madame Grès) – drapes, Nina Ricci – romanticism and Shiaparelli – surrealism.

With the Second World War, the little black dress represented 'the Resistance'. Shortened again for cycling with long sleeves and only a slightly low neckline, in respect for those who were fighting, they were usually made from two or three old ones which had been dyed black and enhanced by a piece of tulle – this being the only fabric which could be found and which was not rationed!

*Didier Ludot is the author of The Little Black Dress, Paris, Assouline 2001.

1955

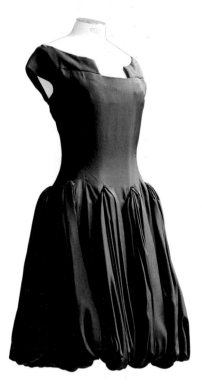

1960

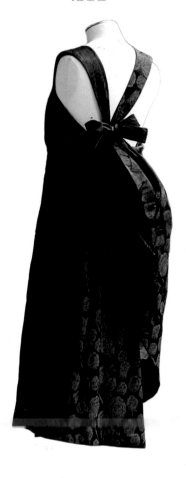

1961

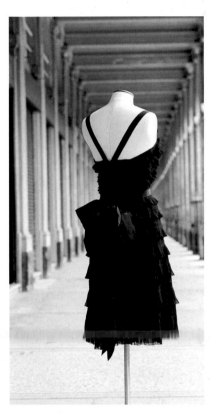

CHRISTIAN DIOR. 1955. AFTERNOON DRESS IN SILK TWILL.
SKIRT WITH PLEATED GODETS.

BALENCIAGA. 1960. EVENING DRESS IN DAMASK SILK.
ASYMMETRIC BACK ACCENTUATED BY A SHELL FORM OF FABRIC.

CHANEL. 1961. DRESS WORN BY DELPHINE SEYRIG IN ALAIN
RESNAIS' *LAST YEAR AT MARIENBAD*. LAYERED BLACK SILK
MUSLIN.

Once the war had finished, the dress became the symbol of existentialism for the 'fairer sex'. It was worn by the zazou-suited 'swingers' before being submerged by the New Look. Reverting back to extreme femininity, it was worn fairly long at calf-length, showing a bit of bust with a flattering wasp-like tailored waist. Whether for cocktails or dinner, it became the apparel of the beautiful, idle rich such as Mona Bismarck and the Duchess of Windsor.

With the 1960s, the advent of the ready-to-wear market and the new wave of cinema, the little black dress became the uniform of the bourgeoisie – simple cuts, straight and democratic.

A string of pearls and a chignon in the nape of the neck, accompanied by a boléro, was a 'must'.

1969

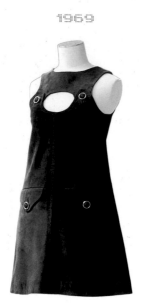

EMANUEL UNGARO. Mini dress in black suede with cut-out keyhole under neckline.

1972

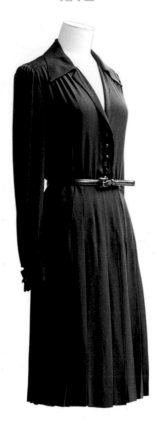

YVES SAINT LAURENT. Crêpe de chine shirtwaister dress. Box pleated at waistband. Style and simplicity combined.

1981

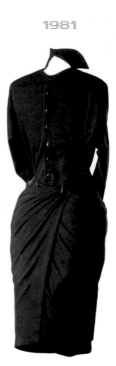

ALAÏA. Jersey wool dress. Gathered apron held by black patent leather belt belonging to the wardrobe of the famous model Bettina.

1983-1984

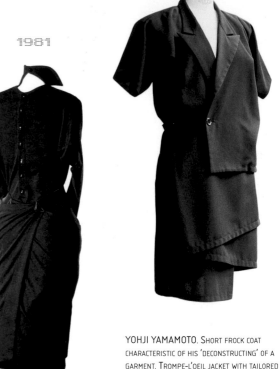

YOHJI YAMAMOTO. Short frock coat characteristic of his 'deconstructing' of a garment. Trompe-l'oeil jacket with tailored collar.

Later on, during the 1968 riots and the 'flower power' era, it was worn as a 'mini' little black dress. Stylish women such as Edmonde Charles-Roux or Françoise Giroud could be seen dancing at Regine's or Castel, wearing Yves Saint Laurent's shirtwaister or Dior's clothing decorated with precious stones. At the beginning of the 1980s, designers such as Alaïa, Mugler and Montana followed suit using more figure-hugging fabrics with padded shoulders. Marked tailoring and teetering on high heels, the Parisian black dress stood its ground as the wave of Japanese designers such as Issey Miyake, Rei Kawakubo and Yohji Yamamoto swept through the capital.

1992

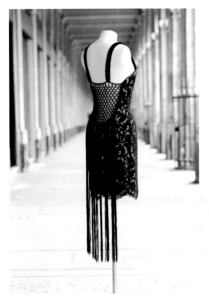

CHRISTIAN LACROIX. COCKTAIL DRESS IN ABSINTHE GREEN DUCHESS SATIN OVERLAID WITH A BLACK MACHINE EMBROIDERED LACE. MACRAMÉ BACK WITH LONG FRINGES.

2003

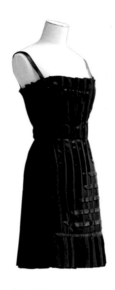

LANVIN BY ALBER ELBAZ. PLEATED DRESS DECORATED IN FRONT WITH SATIN RIBBONS.

2006

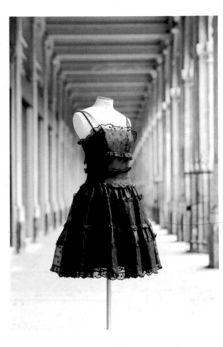

2006 DIDIER LUDOT. 'GRAND ALIBI' MODEL FROM A COLLECTION DESIGNED AS A HOMAGE TO THE ELEGANCE OF HITCHCOCK'S HEROINES. ORGANDY EMBROIDERED WITH SPOTS.

It also made a remarkable come-back to the haute-couture scene following the advent of Karl Lagerfield with Chanel as well as Christian Lacroix, whose fashion house was established in 1987. The 1990s were black, however, the little black dress made from nylon and worn with a Prada belt, held its own in amongst what was essentially a sombre wardrobe. Revered by new designers ranging from Margiela to Helmut Lang, or the minimalist Antwerp group and its 'destruction', it managed to maintain its position with the decadent, almost indecent, designs of Alexander McQueen and Galliano for Dior.

By the end of the 20th century and the beginning of the 21st, it was capable of turning heads again with the dramatic designs of Viktor & Rolf and Alber Elbaz for Lanvin. For this free spirit, which no couturier will ever be able to appropriate, still epitomises eternal femininity.

Redolent of elegance and the French socio-political revolution for almost 80 years, the little black dress has become an obligatory exercise for every designer or couturier as every American client pursues their quest for the symbol of elegance and Parisian style.

Definition by Lutz

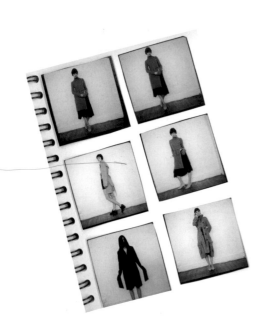

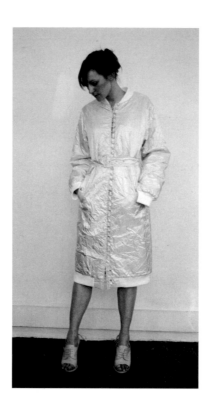

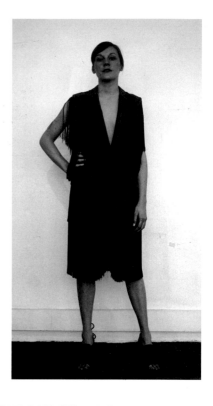

EXTRACT FROM LUTZ'S NOTEBOOK PRESENTING DIFFERENT LOOKS FOR THE AUTUMN-WINTER 2004 AND SPRING-SUMMER 2005 COLLECTIONS.

BOMBER JACKETS – FEMININE NEW LOOK. BOMBER JACKET REWORKED INTO A DRESS-COAT WITH A SERIES OF COVERED BUTTONS USING LOOP FASTENINGS, A PARTICULARLY FEMININE FINISHING DETAIL.

DOUBLE BREASTED JACKET – FLOWING NEW LOOK. MAN'S JACKET REWORKED INTO A DRESS WITH FRINGES. THE SLEEVES HAVE BEEN REMOVED TO FEMINISE THE MODEL. THE CHOICE OF COLOURFUL FRINGES GIVES A TOUCH OF FANTASY TO A SOMBRE JACKET: THE SUIT IS TRANSFORMED INTO A FLUID PRODUCT.

To illustrate the notion of the new look we have chosen the work of the young designer Lutz. His collections demonstrate the possibilities of changing the original clothing model around.

The new look works on ambiguity, it awakens a vague memory of something … it is primarily a subtle reworking of a garment with the aim of keeping its identity.

The starting point of a new look item requires some careful studying. For example, the question needs to be asked as to what makes a garment a basic item, otherwise known as a classic, timeless and forever fashionable wardrobe item? It seems that it is essential because it has a reason for being there: the reefer jacket, the straight skirt and jeans, for example, have generation after generation, remained indispensable items of clothing. The classic's useful characteristic constitutes the foundation of the work. To create a new look product, it is a question of observing how our everyday lives evolve and to make the original garment evolve accordingly.

Nowadays a well-conceived garment is in fact a hybrid of some-

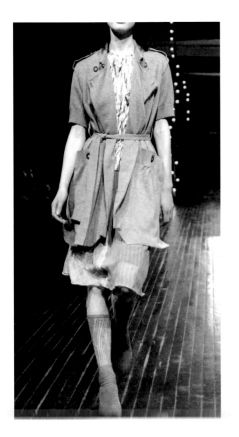

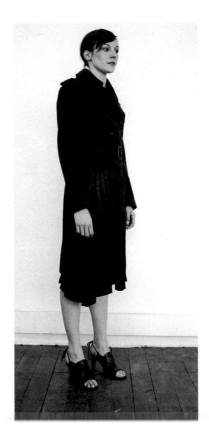

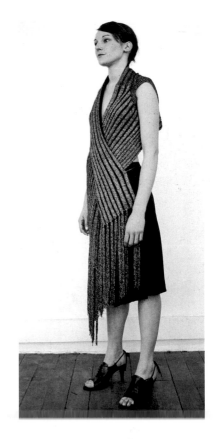

KNITTED TRENCH COAT – NEW FABRIC. USING A KNITTED
FABRIC GIVES THIS TRENCH COAT A SOFT 'CARDIGAN' FEEL.

TAIL COAT TRENCH COAT – FEMININE NEW LOOK. A TAIL
COAT REDINGOTE/RIDING JACKET REWORKED AS A TRENCH COAT
MAKING A HYBRID GARMENT.

FEMININE SCARF – NEWSTYLING. VERY LONG LUREX
KNITTED SCARF TRANSFORMED INTO A JACKET. CROSSED IN THE
FRONT AND TIED AT THE BACK.

thing which follows our daily rhythms, suitable for every occasion and above all, versatile. An example of this is Coco Chanel who famously adapted a man's tweed jacket and tailored it for women.

I have worked with the tail coat in this way for the image it evokes is one of immediate ambivalence.

Another principle of the remake is the reversal of values. For example, it is possible to lose the virile characteristic of a military uniform by adding very feminine details and modifying their proportions. It then becomes a completely new and different product just by adding a feminine aspect to a masculine base. The public is surprised yet finds a point of reference by recognising the garment's origins. It is the same thing with fabrics and emblems: a biker's leather jacket made in braided tweed can become a couture item whilst an Yves Saint Laurent suit, made from denim with stitching and zip fastenings, can become a high street product.

The gesture or the way in which a garment is worn can also suggest an interesting type of 'freeze-frame' interpretation – for example when a shawl is fixed as a jacket.

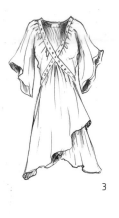
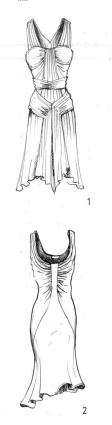
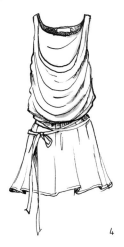
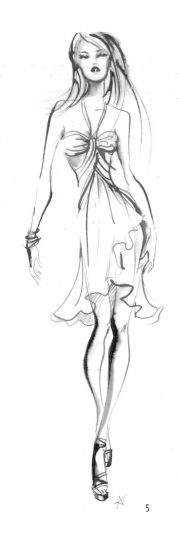

'DRESS' SHOPPING

1. Dress draped in front with a rounded low neckline and asymmetric flares.
2. Draped bustier dress in jersey silk.
3. Cross-heart dress with embroidered edging.
4. Short sleeveless tee-shirt dress with hipster belt.
5. Bustier dress cut away below bust with asymmetric flares.

Shopping is the study of current fashion enabling the designer to ascertain seasonal trends and their evolution in relation to the previous seasons. It consists of finding a selection of the 'best-of' silhouettes and themes which offer an overview of what is available on the high street.

It is also a means of getting to know the distribution networks better. Every designer must fully understand the market in order to successfully target their product as well as be able to differentiate between luxury items and chain store products. They must also be able to define the products corresponding branch of fashion: for example, each socio-professional category as well as each person and their own definition of fashion in relation to their particular taste, place of origin and quality demands.

Shopping also introduces the merchandising aspect into the spectrum. This is an activity which consists of organising a collection as a plan adapted to the market (see pp. 58-9).

With the professional, shopping is almost an automatic reflex. Certain labels integrate this into their forecasting studies. It must not, however, be seen as an excuse for imitation or plagiarism as a lack of creativity can easily lead to the decline of a label.

This activity can also serve as a general observation of the catwalk's influence on the high street. For example, sporting and cultural events can be portrayed in the selections made by the department store buyers when a collection is presented.

Shopping can be organised by product: dresses, blouses or tops, jackets, accessories etc. as well as sub-divisions thereof. For example, in the case of the dress – shirtdress, fitted-dress, dress-coat, sundress .... The research results are sorted by vol-

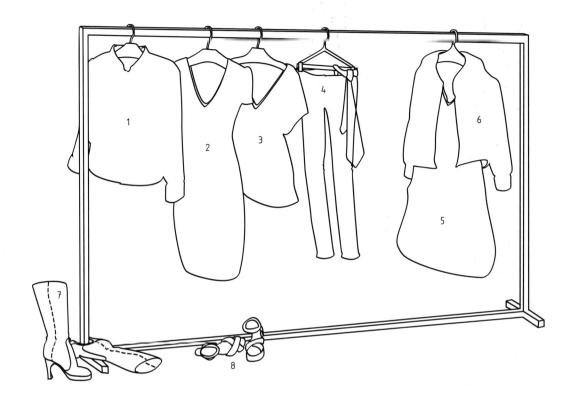

'TREND' SHOPPING: OFFSET THE FEMININE WITH MASCULINE CLOTHING BY WEARING A COUTURE OR VINTAGE ITEM WITH SEPARATES.

1. MAN'S SHIRT (DEPARTMENT STORE, 69 EUROS)
2. VINTAGE DRESS (VINTAGE COUTURE 450 EUROS)
3. LOOSE FITTING BLOUSE (DESIGNER 180 EUROS)
4. A CLASSIC: FITTED JEANS (CLASSIC, 120 EUROS) ACCESSORISE WITH A SCARF
5. SILK DRESS (LUXURY PRÊT-À-PORTER 1,200 EUROS)
6. LEATHER FLYING JACKET (DESIGNER, 520 EUROS)
7. 1970S BOOTS (VINTAGE 110 EUROS)
8. PLATFORM STRAP SANDALS (LUXURY 525 EUROS)

ume (ball, wide, tight-fitting), by colour and by pattern (stripes, dots, squares). Shopping can also be presented under the form of themes or looks, for example, sailor, military, tartan, sport etc.

With the gathering of this information, seasonal details can be noted such as types of shirt sleeves i.e. puffed, ruched, pleated, etc.

Shopping has also created a new metier – that of the private stylist or 'personal shopper' as it is known in the United States. Here the large department stores offer this service to clients who are short on time or do not have the inclination to search through the aisles. This represents a new vision of luxury that the young designer must take on board.

In large department stores such as Selfridges, for example, more and more private stylist salons have been created for those who require this type of personal and professional service. Helmut Lang is a good example of a designer who responded to this type of individual demand with his custom-made garments.

The private stylist's selection must respond to the client's demands swiftly making sure no time is lost or wasted. This metier requires a highly-developed understanding of the fashion culture with all its labels and products as well as an ability to coordinate products and create new looks.

The private stylist's job is similar to that of the photo stylist who works in collaboration with fashion magazine editors and photographers selecting the most interesting items of the season for the collection's presentation.*

*The work of the photo stylist is explained in more detail in an interview with Rebecca Leach (see Chapter 6, pp. 174-5).

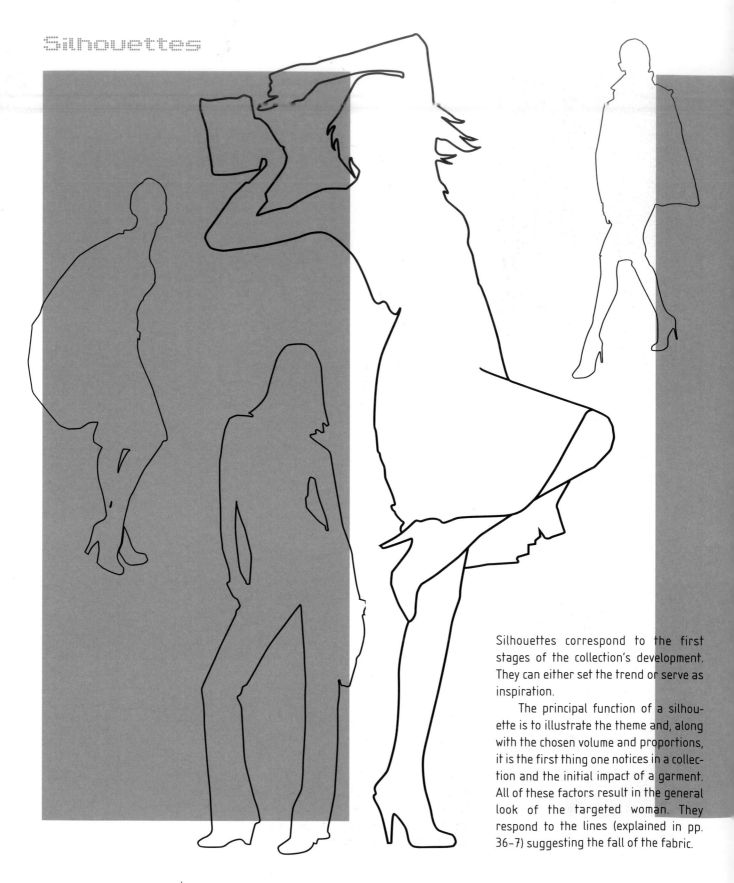

Silhouettes correspond to the first stages of the collection's development. They can either set the trend or serve as inspiration.

The principal function of a silhouette is to illustrate the theme and, along with the chosen volume and proportions, it is the first thing one notices in a collection and the initial impact of a garment. All of these factors result in the general look of the targeted woman. They respond to the lines (explained in pp. 36–7) suggesting the fall of the fabric.

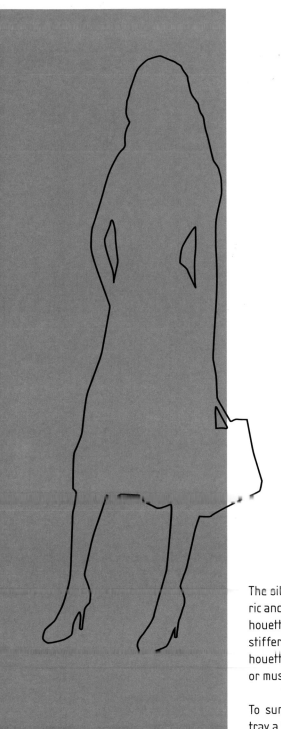

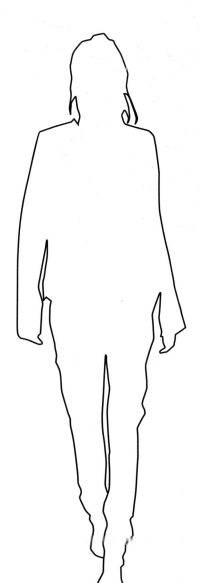

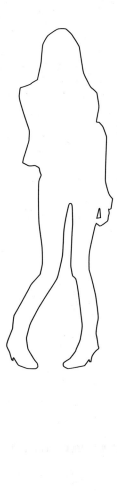

The silhouette governs the choice of fabric and how it will be used: a geometric silhouette for example, will demand more stiffer or rigid fabrics whereas a soft silhouette which would require more crêpes or muslins etc.

To summarise, the silhouette must portray a fragile yet fundamental balance of line, look, proportion and volume as it dictates the general spirit of a collection right from the very beginning.

As with fashion illustrations, but even more so, the silhouette presents the look of a collection. These looks reflect the coordination of the products and, between them, harmonise and illustrate the collection's theme. The number of silhouettes required relates to the amount of passages planned for the fashion show (see Chapter 6, pp. 172–3).

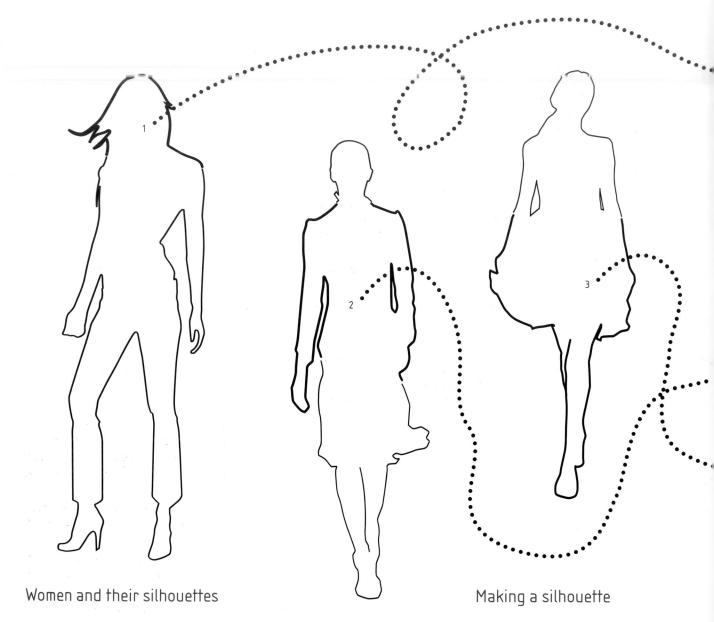

Women and their silhouettes

Each silhouette must represent a particular type of woman. The mythical silhouette of Coco Chanel with her hat and cigarette corresponds to the emancipated and independent woman from between the wars. That of Sonia Rykiel and flamboyant red mane immediately evokes the bohemian artist of 1968. And that of Jean Seberg who seduced the whole of France in Jean-Luc Goddard's *Breathless* (1959) with her short hair and plain clothes which symbolised eternal adolescence. Here we have three silhouettes and already three different types of woman across several decades. A final example is when Yves St. Laurent in 1966 dressed his models in smoking jackets thus creating a new silhouette which corresponded to a type of woman which perhaps Charlotte Rampling epitomised the best.

Making a silhouette

Silhouettes are made, either by drawing with a pencil or felt pen, by cutting out and collage or by tracing. It is a question of gradually building up, by eye, the contours which will constitute the style of the collection. A well-proportioned silhouette illustrates the precision and the correct balance needed for the form and volume. It also indicates how good the designer's eye is.

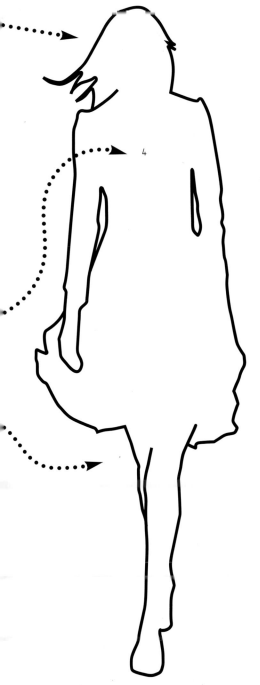

4

COLLAGE.EXAMPLE

1. THE FIRST SILHOUETTE HAS A NATURAL FEEL DUE TO THE MOVE-MENT OF THE HAIR. THIS GIVES THE EFFECT OF A MODERN 'DISCO' STYLE FROM THE POSTURE TO THE ACCESSORIES AND LINE OF THE CLOTHES.

2. THE SECOND SILHOUETTE IS QUITE CLASSIC. THE TAILORING SUG-GESTS AN AUSTERE FEEL.

3. THE THIRD SILHOUETTE EVOKES AN EXUBERANCE WITH ITS BIL-LOWING SKIRT. THE VOLUME OF THE SKIRT CREATES THE IMPRES-SION OF LIGHTNESS AND FEMININITY.

4. THIS SILHOUETTE ECHOES THE FIRST WITH ITS NATURAL HAIR-STYLE, THE STRUCTURE OF THE JACKET FROM THE SECOND GIVING IT A CERTAIN DYNAMISM AND FINALLY THE VOLUMINOUS SKIRT FROM THE THIRD BRINGS A LIGHTNESS AND FEMININITY. A COMBINATION OF THESE THREE GIVES THE OUTFIT A CONTEMPORARY, ORIGINAL FEEL.

Making a silhouette using collage

Collage allows you to fully understand the elaboration or embellishment of a silhouette. Our example shows the work stemming from three different sources of inspiration.

In the case of an historical theme, for example, it will be interesting to combine a top, representing a particular era, with a contemporary bottom and finish it with a hairstyle which defines the desired style of the targeted woman.

Equally, you can compose a sil-houette from abstract images borrowed from architecture like Rei Kawakubo, for example, in his collection 'Comme des Garçons'. They would engender a new style of innovative volume and prop-ortions. Or, quite simply, employ varying cut-out shapes using one or several sheets of paper and basic tools such as glue and scissors.

You can also digitally enhance your ideas using Photoshop as we have done in our example.

Well-conceived silhouettes will help the work of the designer since the choice of fabric and product shapes are already implied in the sketches. The under-standing of the collection will then be made easier for the designer's assistant as well as for the press and clients.

Research drawn from diverse sources of inspiration such as historical, ethnological or even current fashion, will significantly assist elaborating the silhouettes. The proportions of the initial visuals can be thus exaggerated to inform the idea.

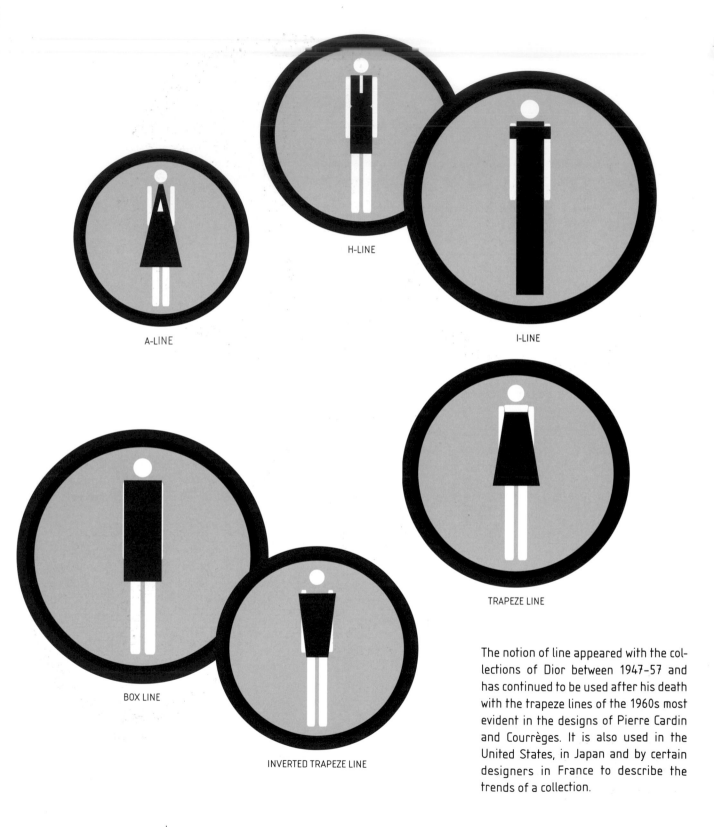

A-LINE

H-LINE

I-LINE

BOX LINE

INVERTED TRAPEZE LINE

TRAPEZE LINE

The notion of line appeared with the collections of Dior between 1947–57 and has continued to be used after his death with the trapeze lines of the 1960s most evident in the designs of Pierre Cardin and Courrèges. It is also used in the United States, in Japan and by certain designers in France to describe the trends of a collection.

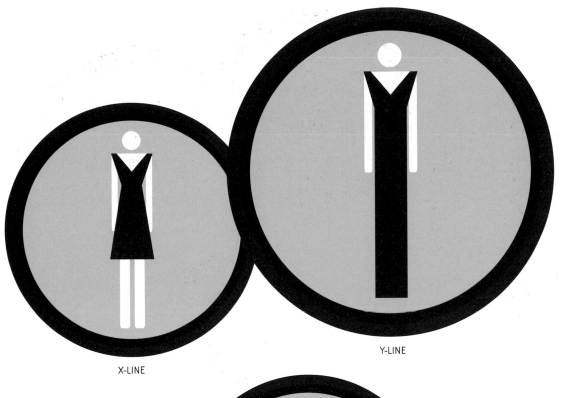

X-LINE

Y-LINE

BALL LINE

OVAL LINE

Today the silhouettes tend to dictate the variety of the creations' shapes but one should be familiar with the official terms. The names of the different lines refer to simple geometric figures or to letters which symbolise the shape and general feeling of the garment.

The most common of these are represented above.

Classic garments are characterised either by their cut or their name. They are products which have endured the ever-evolving fashion trends and global morphology. In relation to the general evolution of women's shapes, varying sizes, age categories or differences in shapes around the world, they still remain easily identifiable.

They fall into two groups:

- Lightweight, dressmaking fabrics, which includes the bodice, the dress, the skirt with their cut variations (straight lines, flared, cut on the bias or draped);
- Tailored, heavier fabrics including the suit, or sleeved item, originating from men's traditional separates or uniforms like jackets and coats.

Knitwear items are distinguished by the fact that they require techniques and specific machines which gives the garments their particular appearance.

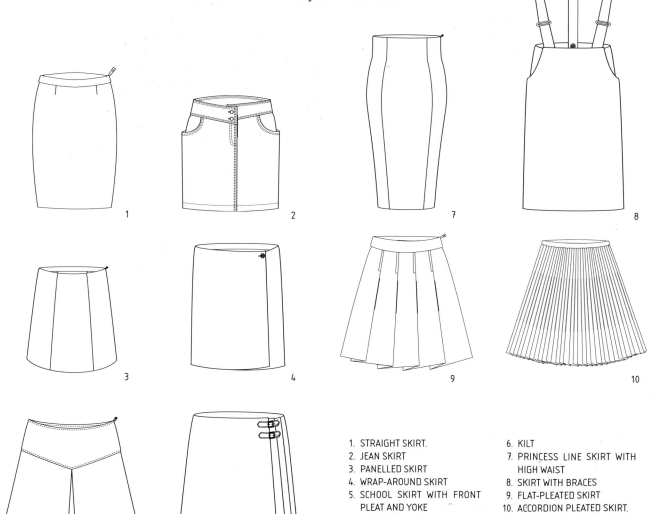

1. STRAIGHT SKIRT.
2. JEAN SKIRT
3. PANELLED SKIRT
4. WRAP-AROUND SKIRT
5. SCHOOL SKIRT WITH FRONT PLEAT AND YOKE
6. KILT
7. PRINCESS LINE SKIRT WITH HIGH WAIST
8. SKIRT WITH BRACES
9. FLAT-PLEATED SKIRT
10. ACCORDION PLEATED SKIRT.

Skirts

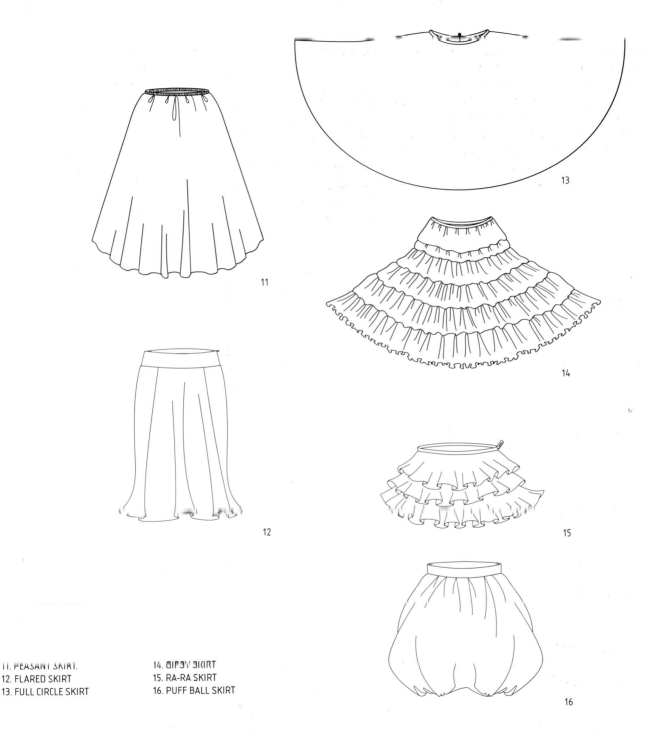

11. PEASANT SKIRT.
12. FLARED SKIRT
13. FULL CIRCLE SKIRT

14. GIPSY SKIRT
15. RA-RA SKIRT
16. PUFF BALL SKIRT

Straight, flared, bias, pleated, gathered, flounced and balloon skirts are all examples of a classic separate. Our selection demonstrates a certain number of timeless cuts which are currently used today. A classic can also be identified by the fabric, details and finishes used, such as overstitching, pockets and fly openings for denim skirts etc. Nevertheless, it will always remain a simple product which is easy to wear.

Dresses

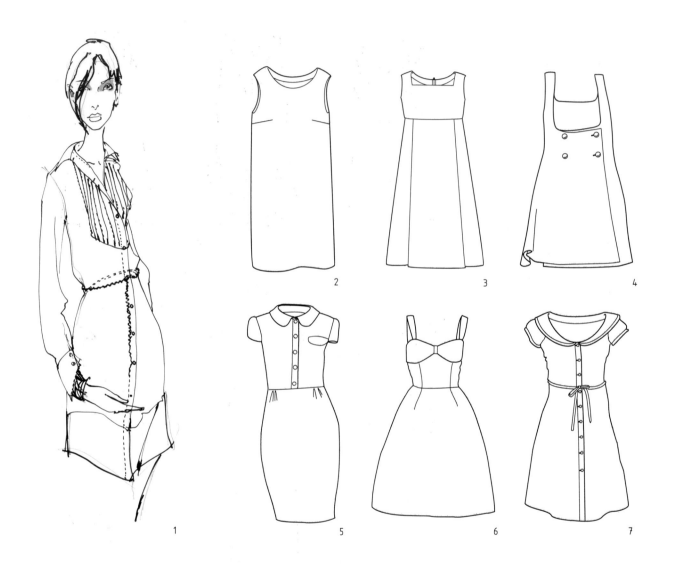

1. SHIRT DRESS WITH PIN STITCHED BIB
2. SHIFT DRESS
3. A-LINE DRESS
4. PINAFORE DRESS
5. POLO DRESS
6. 1950s BUSTIER DRESS
7. ROBE CHEMISIER 1940.

The dress is a one piece garment with or without sleeves. It can be the result of a combination of a top and a skirt, as in the case of bustier dresses and sun dresses (where the skirt is attached to a bra). Our examples of the polo and shirt dress (nos. 1 and 5) are also tailored.

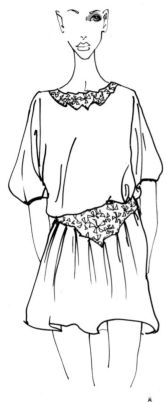

8

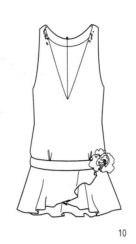

9

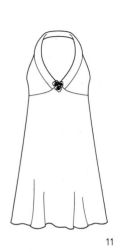

10

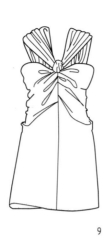

11

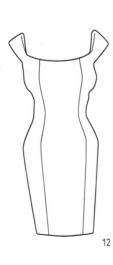

12

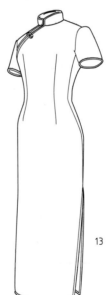

13

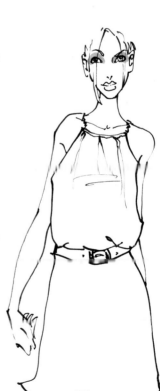

14

8. TUNIC DRESS
9. DRAPED DRESS
10. FLAPPER DRESS
11. SUN DRESS

12. SHEATH OR PRINCESS LINE DRESS.
13. CHINESE INSPIRED DRESS
14. HALTER NECK DRESS -- BILLOWING AT THE WAIST

Trousers

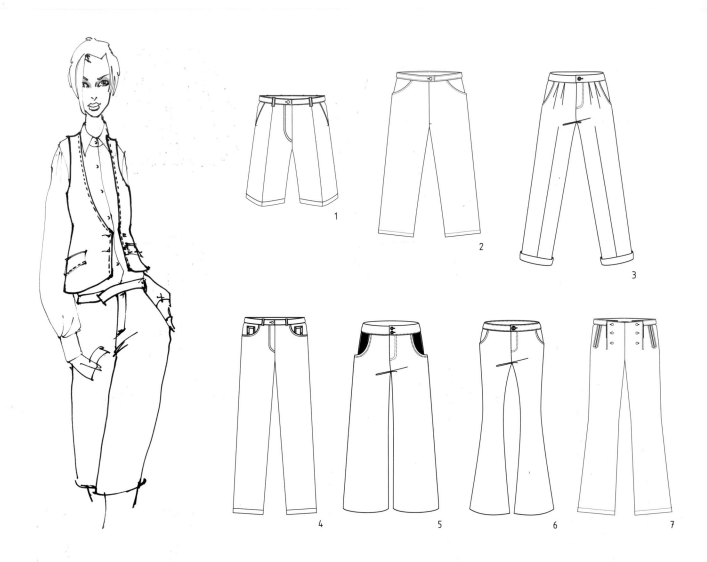

1
2
3
4
5
6
7

Originally trousers were a tight-fitting, knee-length masculine garment, worn with underwear, by nobles, and without, by peasants.

After the French Revolution, long trousers were adopted by every man, being made from fine fabrics, such as wool, for the bourgeoisie and from coarser, more hard-wearing fabrics for the working classes.

Foreign sources also exist such as the *saroual* which was a traditional garment worn as a uniform by the Algerian light infantry corps, known as the *zouaves* in 1830.

Trousers became unisex in the 20th century.

These separates are defined by length, width, details (pleats, folds, gathers, drawstring belts, pockets, flies/zips, and turn-ups) and by the position of the belt (high, low, drop or fitted waist).

The shape of the trouser often corresponds to the original usage:
• military (combat pants, sailors trousers)
• sportswear (jodhpurs, tracksuits)
• utilitarian (butchers' and mechanics' overalls, boiler suits)

CHAPTER 1
Products

1. BERMUDA SHORTS
2. CROPPED TROUSERS
3. CLASSIC TROUSERS WITH PLEATS AND TURN-UPS
4. 5-POCKETED MEN'S JEANS
5. BELL-BOTTOM TROUSERS
6. FLARES
7. SAILORS' TROUSERS
8. JODHPURS
9. BLOOMER
10. SAROUAL
11. DUNGAREES
12. OVERALL OR JUMPSUIT
13. BAGGY COMBAT TROUSERS
14. TRACKSUIT
15. SKI PANTS

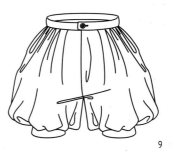

9

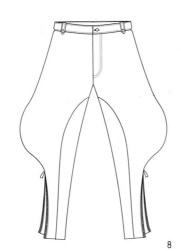

8

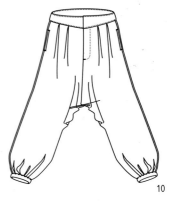

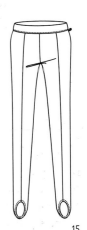

10

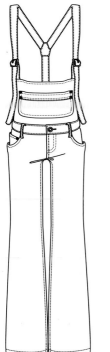

11

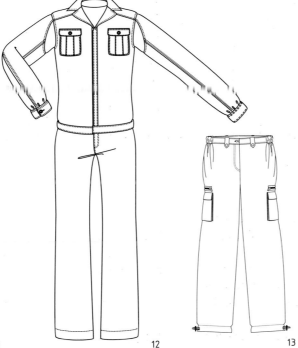

12

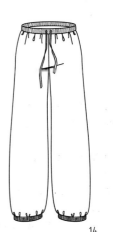

13

14

15

Jackets

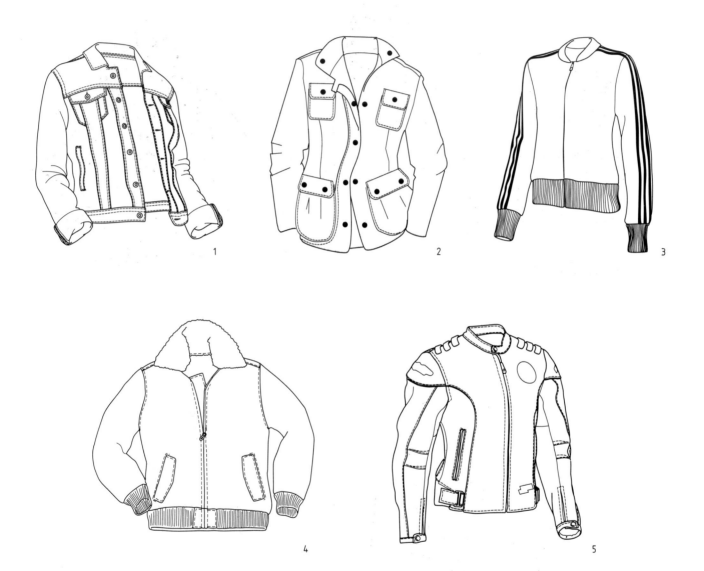

1

2

3

4

5

Jackets are items borrowed from the male wardrobe. The conception and manufacture of the sleeves, armholes and linings which make the structure of the garment (cloth, epaulettes, shoulder padding etc.) require a particular type of care and precision.

They usually originate from military, sport or ethnic (parkas) clothing. The choice of fabrics linked to the model's style is relatively fixed: leather for motorcycle jackets, jean/denim material for Levi style cuts etc.

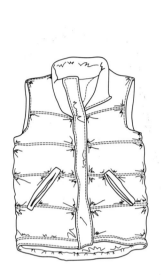

6

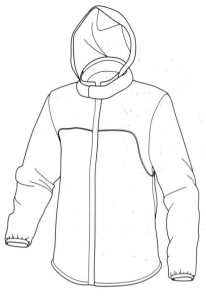

7

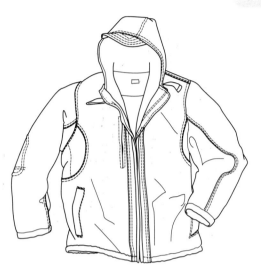

8

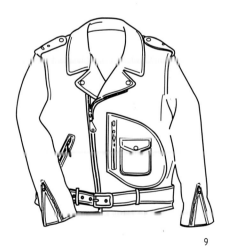

9

1 JEAN JACKET
2. HUNTING JACKET
3. TRACKSUIT TOP
4. BOMBER JACKET
5. BIKERS' JACKET
6. SLEEVELESS PUFFA OR QUILTED
   JACKET
7. PARKA
8. WINDCHEATER/ANORAK
9. AVIATOR OR FLYING JACKET

Tailored jackets

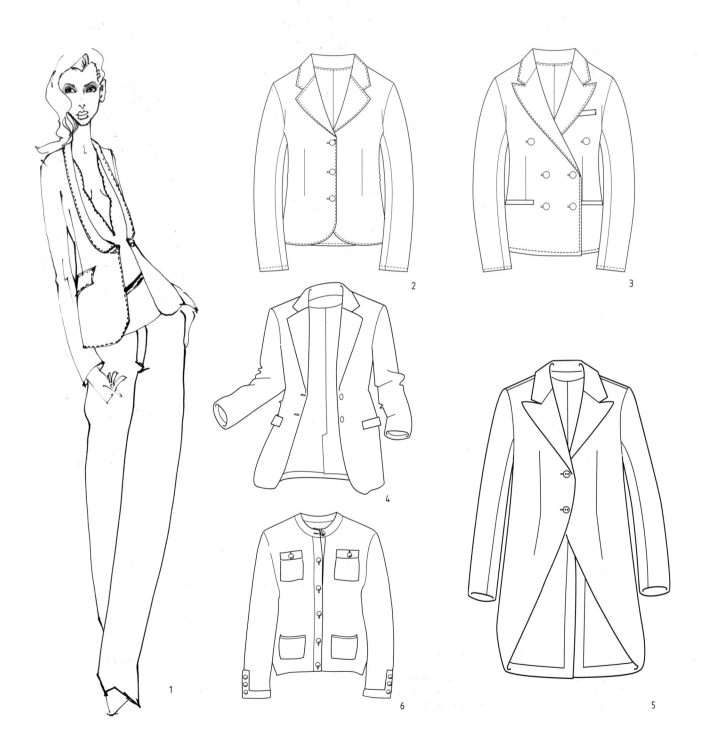

1

2

3

4

5

6

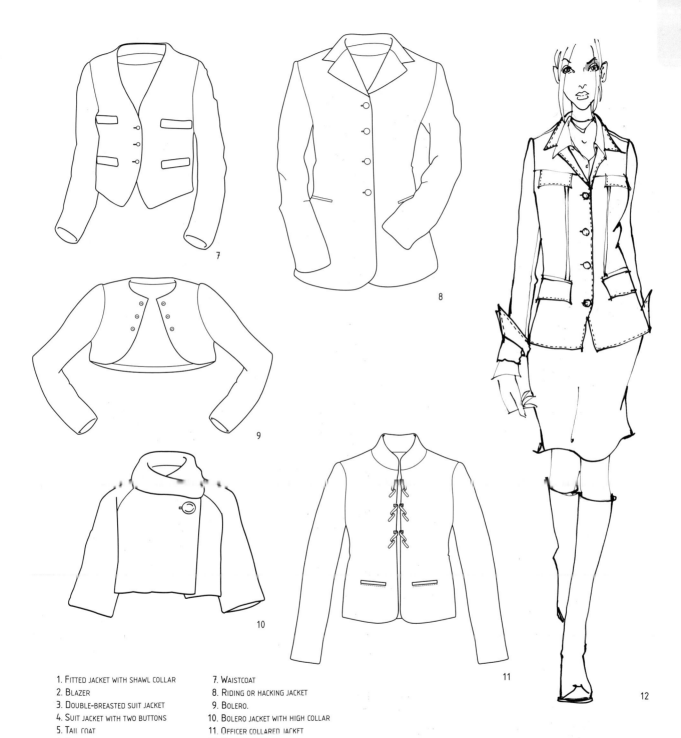

1. FITTED JACKET WITH SHAWL COLLAR
2. BLAZER
3. DOUBLE-BREASTED SUIT JACKET
4. SUIT JACKET WITH TWO BUTTONS
5. TAIL COAT
6. CHANEL SUIT
7. WAISTCOAT
8. RIDING OR HACKING JACKET
9. BOLERO.
10. BOLERO JACKET WITH HIGH COLLAR
11. OFFICER COLLARED JACKET
12. SAFARI JACKET

Coats

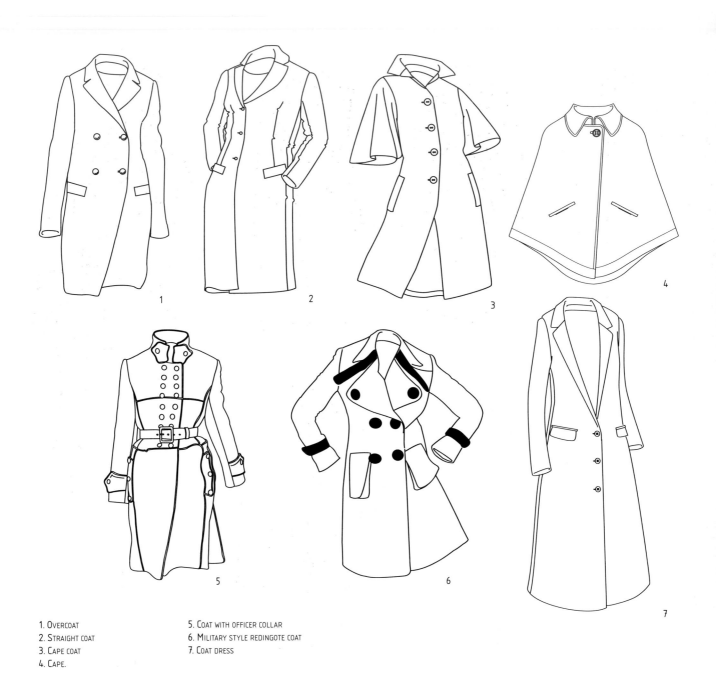

1. OVERCOAT
2. STRAIGHT COAT
3. CAPE COAT
4. CAPE.

5. COAT WITH OFFICER COLLAR
6. MILITARY STYLE REDINGOTE COAT
7. COAT DRESS

Coat shapes are also derived from the male wardrobe and most often from the military wardrobe.

Coats main function is to provide protection against the elements: the waterproof for rain, the woollen coat for the cold, the reefer jacket for the wind (it was used as a windcheater by sailors). The fabric used was determined by its usage. Today, the shape of the coat is more a question of style and they are made in a variety of materials, for example, the knitted trench coat from the Lutz collection presented on page 29.

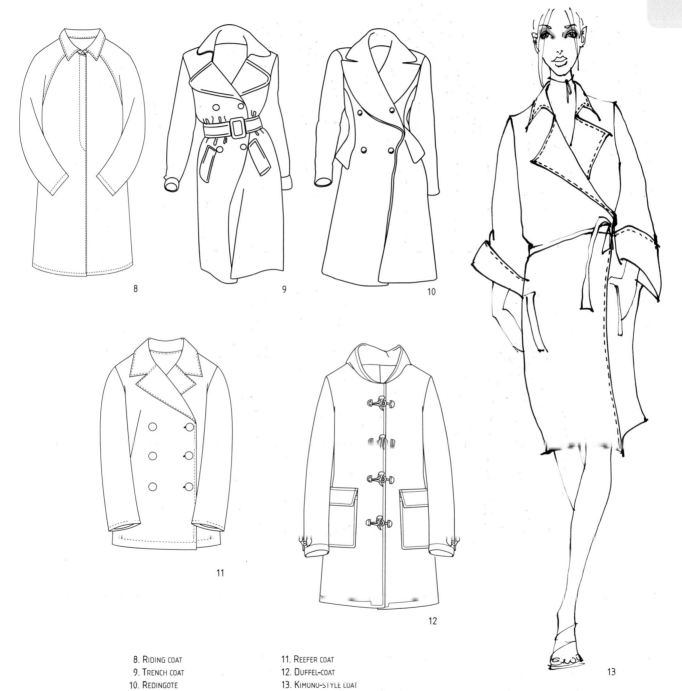

8. RIDING COAT
9. TRENCH COAT
10. REDINGOTE

11. REEFER COAT
12. DUFFEL-COAT
13. KIMONO-STYLE COAT

Knitwear

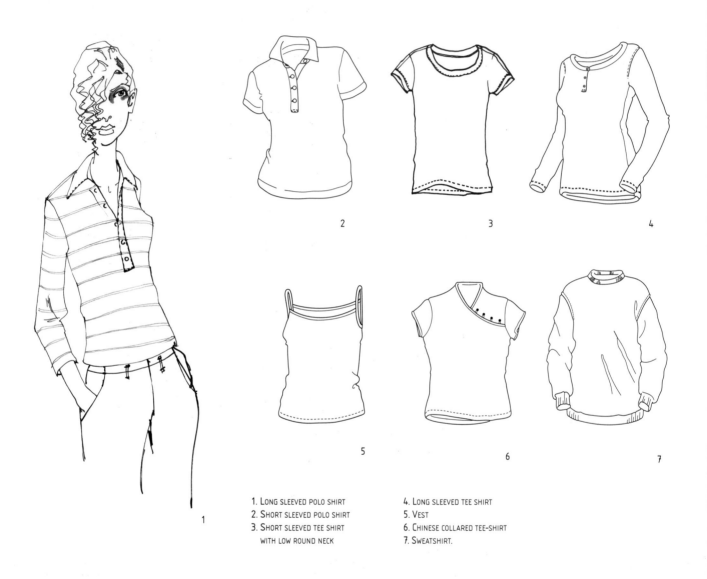

1. LONG SLEEVED POLO SHIRT
2. SHORT SLEEVED POLO SHIRT
3. SHORT SLEEVED TEE SHIRT
   WITH LOW ROUND NECK

4. LONG SLEEVED TEE SHIRT
5. VEST
6. CHINESE COLLARED TEE-SHIRT
7. SWEATSHIRT.

It is important to distinguish between knitwear and 'cut-and-sew' tee-shirt material for sweaters. The latter is knitted industrially on large rolls then cut, like material, with the aid of card patterns (such as jersey, which is worked with thinner or thicker thread, or yarn, for tee-shirts and sweatshirts). In the case of the sweater, the fabric is knitted by machine or by hand allowing direct production of garments such as jumpers, waistcoats etc. The thickness of the garment depends as much on the gauge of the machine as on the type of thread used.

Knitwear requires specific technical knowledge concerning the variety of stitches and finishing which determine the look of the garment. This is why our selection includes variants on collars and products representative of these separates.

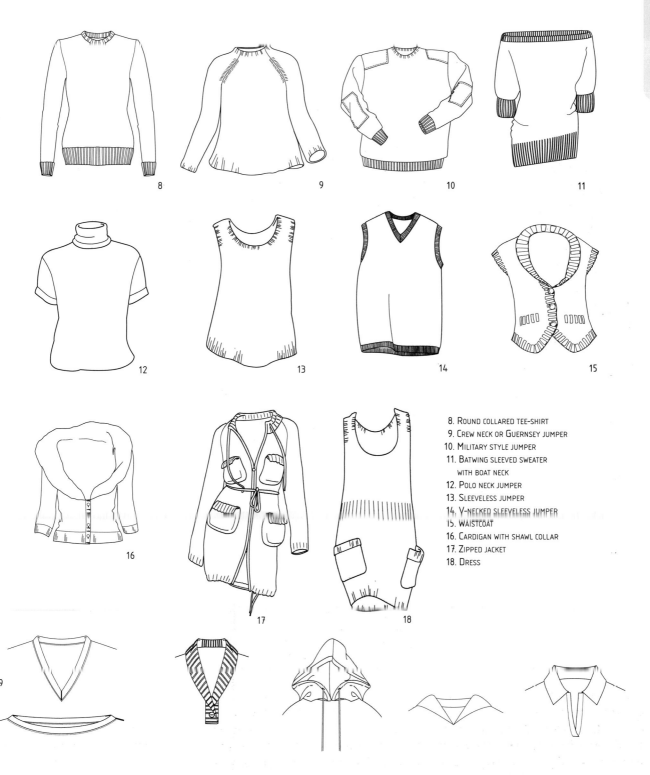

8. ROUND COLLARED TEE-SHIRT
9. CREW NECK OR GUERNSEY JUMPER
10. MILITARY STYLE JUMPER
11. BATWING SLEEVED SWEATER
   WITH BOAT NECK
12. POLO NECK JUMPER
13. SLEEVELESS JUMPER
14. V-NECKED SLEEVELESS JUMPER
15. WAISTCOAT
16. CARDIGAN WITH SHAWL COLLAR
17. ZIPPED JACKET
18. DRESS

19. COLLAR VARIATIONS. FROM LEFT TO RIGHT: V-NECK, BOAT NECK, SHAWL COLLAR, HOOD, SAILOR'S COLLAR, POLO COLLAR WITHOUT BUTTONS

Shirts/blouses

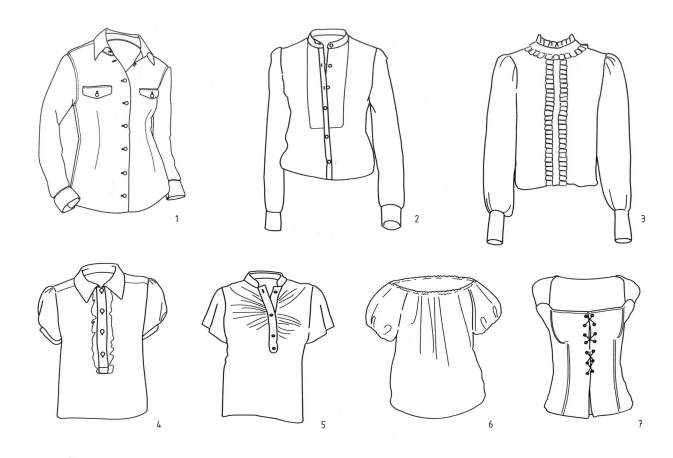

1. CLASSIC SHIRT
2. BLOUSE WITH MILITARY STYLE COLLAR AND PLASTRON.
3. BLOUSE BUTTONED UP THE BACK WITH FULL SLEEVES OVER THE CUFF
4. POLO BLOUSE
5. SHORT SLEEVED BLOUSE WITH MANDARIN COLLAR
6. BOAT NECK BLOUSE
7. BUSTIER BLOUSE

The shirt is one of the oldest items of clothing in the West. Its first appearance was in 5th century BC with the Greeks and subsequently with the Romans (*la tunica*).

For a long time it was worn as an undergarment, by women as well as men, and only became part of men's clothing in 15th century where it discreetly appeared above the vest. In the 19th century, it was still worn with a jacket and was fairly well worked with pleats and bib following the billowing lace of the 17th and 18th centuries. One can see this in illustrations from that period worn by women in side-saddle riding habits.

The evolution concerning the details of sleeves, cuffs and collars enable us to place it in history. For example: Louis XIV sleeves which have been shortened by three rows of billowing gathers and tied up by bows and ribbons, Musketeer cuffs, Danton collars etc.

The shirt took on a new identity with African and Hawaiian prints and the American cowboy flannel check shirts, as well as the heavy woollen ones of Canada. It had, up until then, remained white like the undergarments it was derived from. The introduction of the modern pockets were borrowed from British colonial troops.

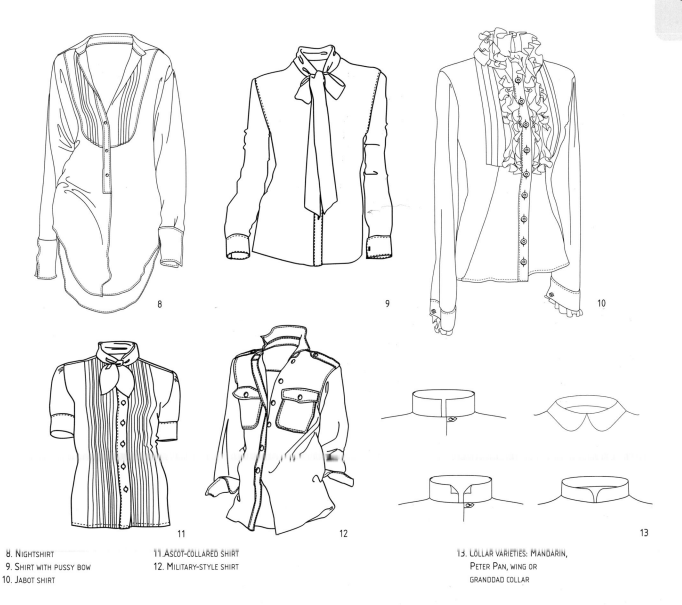

8. NIGHTSHIRT
9. SHIRT WITH PUSSY BOW
10. JABOT SHIRT

11. ASCOT-COLLARED SHIRT
12. MILITARY-STYLE SHIRT

13. COLLAR VARIETIES: MANDARIN,
    PETER PAN, WING OR
    GRANDDAD COLLAR

One can distinguish the woman's blouse, or bodice, which buttoned up the front and was inherited from the shirt worn under a corset, from the blouse which came from the working woman's shirt. The latter being fuller and often buttoning up the back (see illustration no. 3).

For this specific product, it is important to know the principles of the conception and manufacture of collars, sleeves, cuffs, and buttonholing in the front for the man's shirt.

The cuts and finishes are generally over-sewn, but men's shirts can take on the appearance of American tailoring (reversible or over-sewn as with jeans) to give the impression of a sport style.

DRESS FINISHES

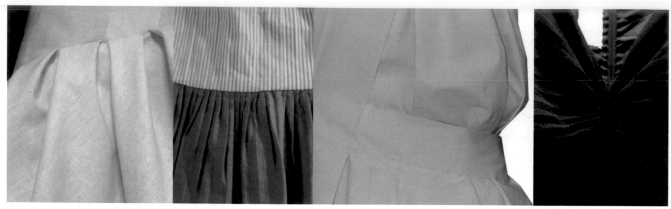

ROUND PLEATS　　　FLAT MINI-PLEAT　　　LARGE PLEATS IN A FITTED WAISTBAND　　　ACCORDION PLEATS

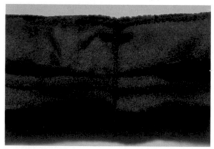

SEWN IN FLAT MINI-PLEATS

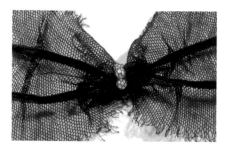

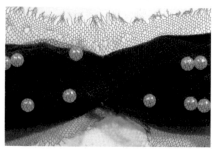

TULLE BOWS WITH PEARLS

The general line and balance of volume are the first things that we notice about a garment, then we look more closely at the detail and finishes. These are often the deciding factor on whether we choose a particular item above another as they determine its originality and quality.

With thorough research afforded to details and finishes, the stylist is able to give a coherence to his or her collection (see 'Ideas Compilations' in the following pages). As with the theme, preliminary research for them originates from a variety of sources. In fact, they must be considered at the outset of the project and be completely integrated into the sketches at the beginning: being added as an after-thought can alter the general balance of a garment and upset the planning of the brand. This, in turn, will compromise the presentation dates, manufacture and delivery.

However, it is necessary to identify the pieces during the fashion shows which have been simplified in a way which responds to the commercial demands of standardising a garment.

A stylist must have a good understanding of the different types of materials, the production tools and the manufacturing constraints for these details and finishes. Moreover, he or she must never lose sight of their functional aspect, particularly with openings and fastenings.

Warp and weft products, made from non-stretch materials, will require openings so that they can be passed over the head and wrists for a shirt, and at the waist for a skirt or trousers etc. These details can be classic, or worked, using particular techniques for hidden buttoning, additions etc.

The comfort of a garment must also be taken into consideration. This is done by creating pleats for ease, for example, by introducing them in the back, up to the shoulder, for men's shirts and in the front, over the chest, for women. All types of pleats, tucks and fittings at the waist are equally indispensable. For even more comfort several materials now include Lycra thread.

Originality in knitwear remains essentially in the finishes. These are techniques such as ribbing which renders the garment more or less stretchy. The types of stitches and threads used will determine its volume, fall and look.

POCKETS

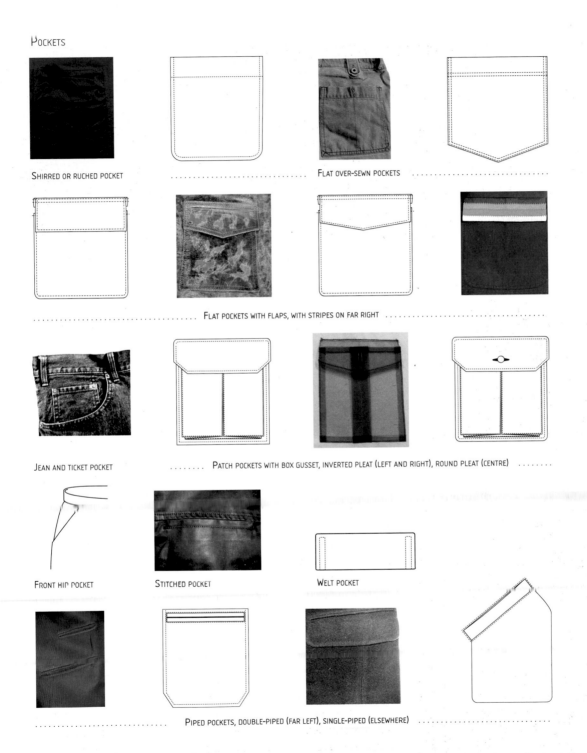

SHIRRED OR RUCHED POCKET . . . . FLAT OVER-SEWN POCKETS . . . .

. . . . FLAT POCKETS WITH FLAPS, WITH STRIPES ON FAR RIGHT . . . .

JEAN AND TICKET POCKET . . . . PATCH POCKETS WITH BOX GUSSET, INVERTED PLEAT (LEFT AND RIGHT), ROUND PLEAT (CENTRE) . . . .

FRONT HIP POCKET   STITCHED POCKET   WELT POCKET

. . . . PIPED POCKETS, DOUBLE-PIPED (FAR LEFT), SINGLE-PIPED (ELSEWHERE) . . . .

It is important to bear in mind that a well-conceived garment adapts itself to different postures. Pockets which are too small or badly placed, for example, are not practical, costly to make and do not necessarily give an originality to a piece of clothing.

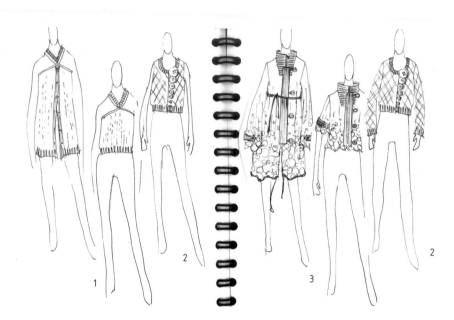

KNITWEAR VARIATIONS 1: COLLAR VARIATIONS 2: ROUND COLLAR VARIATIONS, WAISTCOATS WITH OR WITHOUT SLEEVES 3: LENGTH VARIATIONS AROUND MOTIF, BUTTONING AND UP-TURNED COLLAR.

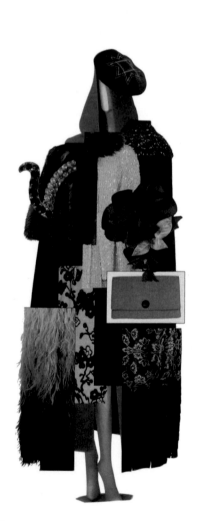

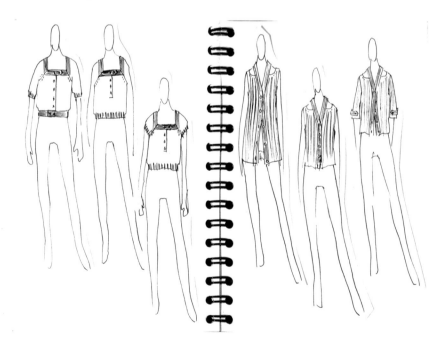

PRODUCTION ON A MANNEQUIN, SHOWING THE OVERALL FEEL OF THE FABRICS OF THE COLLECTION. THE SILHOUETTE, THE HARMONY AND PATTERN COLOURS ARE IMMEDIATELY UNDERSTOOD.

SWEATER VARIATIONS AROUND A SQUARE NECKLINE WITH POLO TRIMMING AND DIFFERING SLEEVES.

LENGTH VARIATIONS AROUND A WAISTCOAT FASTENING, RIBBED FINISH USING STRAPS, ON A CARDIGAN WITH OR WITHOUT SLEEVES.

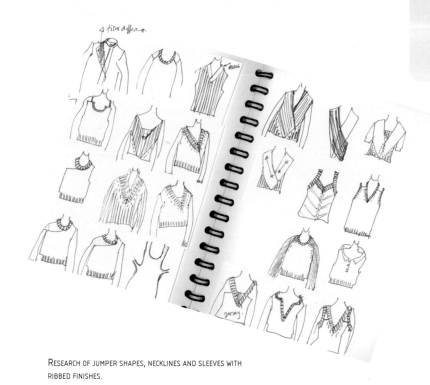

RESEARCH OF JUMPER SHAPES, NECKLINES AND SLEEVES WITH
RIBBED FINISHES.

The compilation of ideas is fundamentally a research of developments from different pieces of the collection using different finishes and original details. And from this, only the best propositions will be kept.

This research can be elaborated by garment (i.e. skirt, dress, trousers, jacket etc.), by fabric or by pattern. The same pattern, for example, can be diversely interpreted using different techniques such as embroidery, patchwork, hand painting or fabric printing.

The pattern research we have presented on pp. 74-9, which shows the development of a flower motif, offers an example of this type of investigation. We have chosen to illustrate this stage by pulling out a few pages from the sketchbook of the young designer Lutz (already mentioned on pp. 28-9).

As well as the sketch, the tools for this research can be very varied. On the opposite page you will find a presentation mannequin covered in fabric swatches and floral motifs showing an original form of compilation.

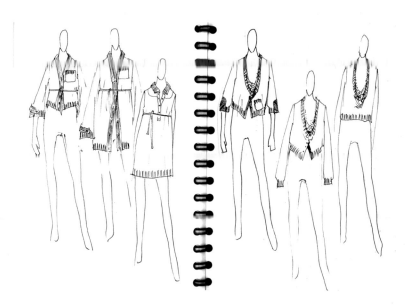

CARDIGAN, LONG WAISTCOAT AND DRESS WITH RIBBED FINISHES
AND TIES UNDER THE BUST.

RESEARCH AROUND A WAISTCOAT AND SLEEVELESS VEST WITH
RIBBED FINISHES.

Collection plan
Lutz, spring-summer collection 2004
Interview with Martine Adrien

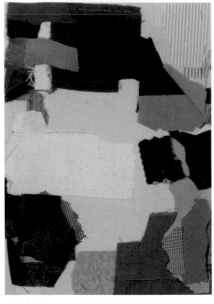

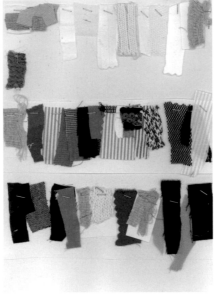

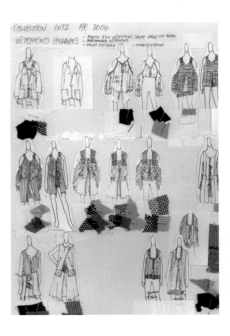

FABRIC CHOICES FOR THE SEASON

FABRIC SELECTION FOR THE ITEMS IN THE COLLECTION COORDINATED BY COLOUR HARMONIES AND PRODUCTS.

COLLECTION PLAN OF 'HYBRID' CLOTHING WITH STRAPS, SHOWING SEVERAL VARIATIONS WITH CORRESPONDING FABRICS.

The collection plan is a very detailed representation of the entire collection, categorised by garments. It must include:

the fashion show items, the look and their accessories
the trademark items destined for the press
the retail outlet items
items destined for overseas clients, categorised by country and world region

The complexity of the above forces the designer to establish a particularly rigorous planning for the collection.

Fashion show organisation

The collection plan lists the items which have to be duplicated for the fashion show by colours and by fabrics, and this, in turn, allows a work plan to be established prior to the manufacture of the pieces. It is a question of finding a balance between these in order to define the looks presented by each theme (see Chapter 6, p. 173).

The collection plan is also indispensable for the organisation of the appearances on the catwalk and it is normally pinned to the wall during the show. It is here where the items are coordinated with their relevant accessories which the model must wear during the presentation and a Polaroid photo captures the desired look (see Chapter 6, p. 184).

Merchandising

The merchandiser plans the season in relation to the results of past seasons and boutique demands. In fact, an item can differ, within the same brand, depending on different countries and

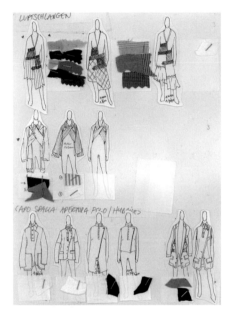

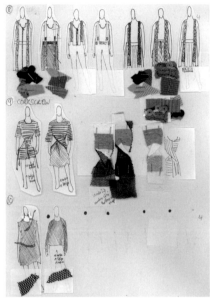

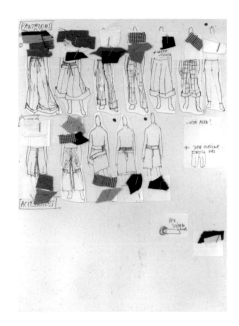

LINE 1: VARIATIONS ON A SKIRT
LINE 2: VARIATIONS ON 'TRENCH' SHIRTS
LINE 3: VARIATIONS ON 'HYBRID' POLOS

LINE 1: VARIATIONS ON A PINAFORE DRESS WITH A TROMPE-L'OEIL EFFECT
LINE 2: OVER-SIZE TEE-SHIRT WITH RIBBED EFFECT
LINE 3: VARIATIONS ON TEE-SHIRT WITH CRISS-CROSS EFFECT

COLLECTION PLAN FOR TROUSERS AND SKIRTS WITH FABRICS.

world regions. For example, for a product such as a dress, a client from Japan and the Asian Pacific region would prefer small, less-fitted dresses, the Americans would prefer more dressy ones and European clients tend to choose printed ones. It is the merchandiser who decides on the products which are essential for sales and coordinates them into the collection plan. Moreover, he, or she, dictates to the designers the important looks and accessories adapted to the brand-targeted clients.

Collection coordinator, Martine Adrien, recalls her experience with Robert Forrest, Ungaro's merchandiser from 1995–2000.

The merchandiser works with a team of designers. After reviewing the results of market research studies, varied and adapted products are required in order to maximise the company's profits.

Therefore, a combination of diverse 'mix and match' items are put forward. Different tops (blouses, sweaters, tank tops etc.) will be associated with different bottoms (skirts, trousers) in coordinating fabrics; for example, bermuda shorts, trousers and a skirt will be proposed for the same top.

Regarding different body shapes, the products' proportions will need to be reconsidered for certain markets, as with that of Japan, which can lead to a complete reinterpretation of the collection's initial plans.

Consumer habits is also a factor which needs to be taken into account. The Japanese and Americans are keener on branding (designer clothing), whereas the English prefer vintage as well as branding.

In the textile world, it is hard to address colour without taking into account whether the fabric is to be dyed or printed. The nature of the fabric and the yarn used, play an all important role in the execution of the colours. The luminosity of the fibre, for example, shiny in the case of silk and matt in that of linen, will modify considerably the perception that one has of the same colour depending on which fabric is used.

As with fabrics, colours are affected by trends, the evolution of ways of life and technological progress within the textile industry.

To imagine a colour range and to organise the fabric swatches in correlation with the themes chosen for a collection involves using a selection of yarns and fabrics proposed by the manufacturers. Today, the advanced technology within the fabric industry allows manufacturers to respond easily to the demands of the fashion designers. However, this is not always without constraints and the minimum quantities imposed for fabrics or original colours can pose high costs for many fashion companies.

Apart from knowing essential technical aspects of how a fabric is manufactured (such as, understanding the nature of the fibres from which it is made, the type of thread torsion, the differing techniques used for fabric making i.e. woven, or not, in the case of knitwear or felt), it is important to know manufacturing cycles and to present, to the professionals, the raw materials from which the product is made, in order to determine a *modus operandi*.

The yearly plan for a fashion designer is also governed by

Chapter 2 - Colours and fabrics

two very important periods, February-March and September, when the large textile fairs such as Première Vision, Exporit, le Cuir in Paris and Texworld take place. This is where selection takes place for the fabrics destined for the collection or for the products in the diffusion lines.

This selection will have an effect, ultimately, on the composition of the colour range, which must correlate with the fabric swatches, if necessary. Conversely, however, it is not unusual to propose the colour range first which, in turn, will direct the final choice of fabrics. This can reduce the amount of constraints right from the beginning of the creative process.

The pattern idea, textile printing and creation of the fabrics for a fabric manufacturer or for specific products in a studio, is

the job of the colourist and the modelmaker. In the studio, they will be able to imagine the original patterns for a collection or for particular accessory lines, in the approximate colour ranges supplied according to the particular print or weave to be used.

In this chapter some fundamental notions are explained concerning the use of colour in fashion. By way of example, a selection of fabrics in relation with different garments are described, as are the methods of pattern development and textile design. It serves as an introduction to this subject as the techniques of textile design require a much deeper understanding of fabrics in general, which cannot be summarised in just a few pages. However, 'fabrics' are discussed in greater detail in a forthcoming *Studies in Fashion* book (*Fabrics and Trends*).

Colours

The use of colour in the fashion world follows the same elementary rules as it does in the graphic arts. For its theoretical aspects, we refer to the colour treatise* defined by Johannes Itten, who was a professor at the Bauhaus between 1919 and 1923. It was he who defined the 12 sections of the colour wheel and it equally known for his description of the principal colour contrasts.

Colours used in fashion are however, very specific. They are different to those used in furnishing. A beautiful colour range in fashion is appropriate to the garment it is intended

for. For example, pastel colours are easily associated with lingerie and baby clothes; darker colours with winter; bright colours with summer and children; metallic and shiny colours with evening wear and fluorescent colours with the sport. This very simplified classification of colour by product is still pertinent today.

Certain colours are so strong that they themselves become the label's identity, for example, Lanvin's blue or Hermès' orange.

PALETTE

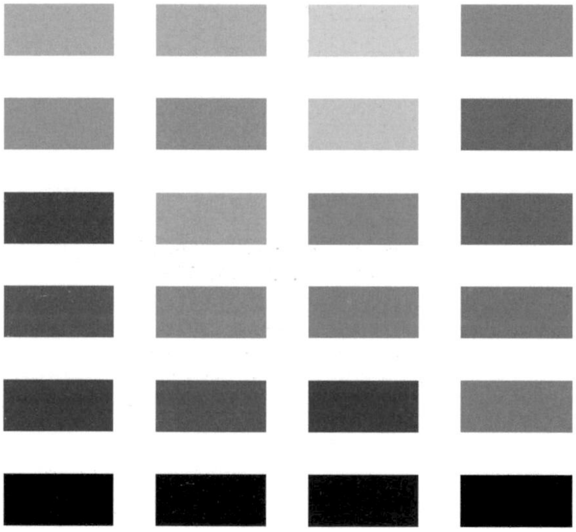

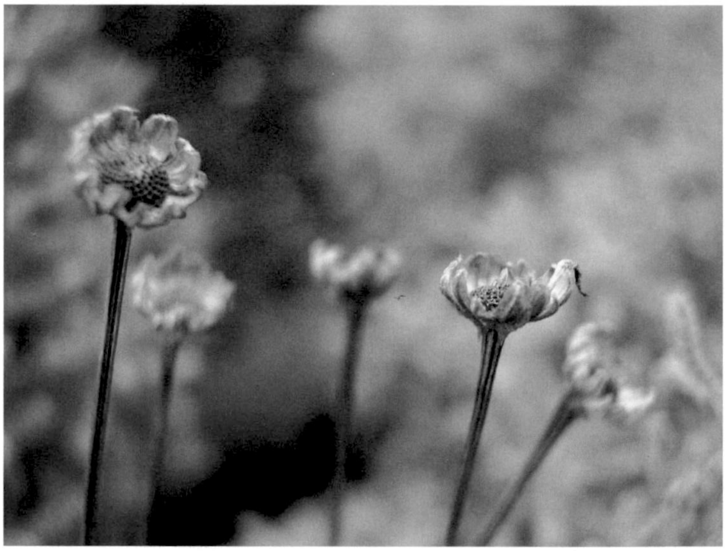

HARMONY

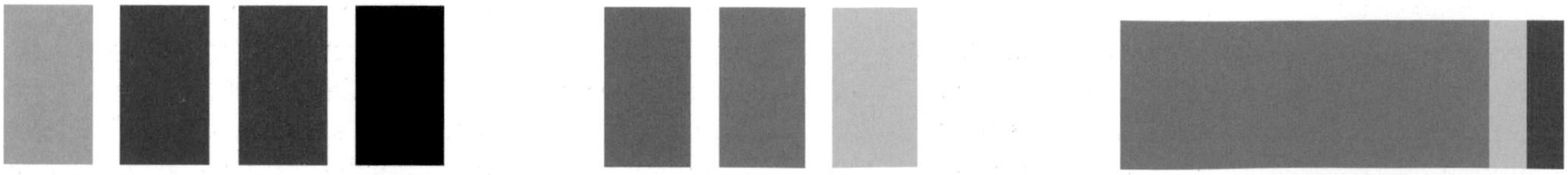

*Art and colour', published in 1961

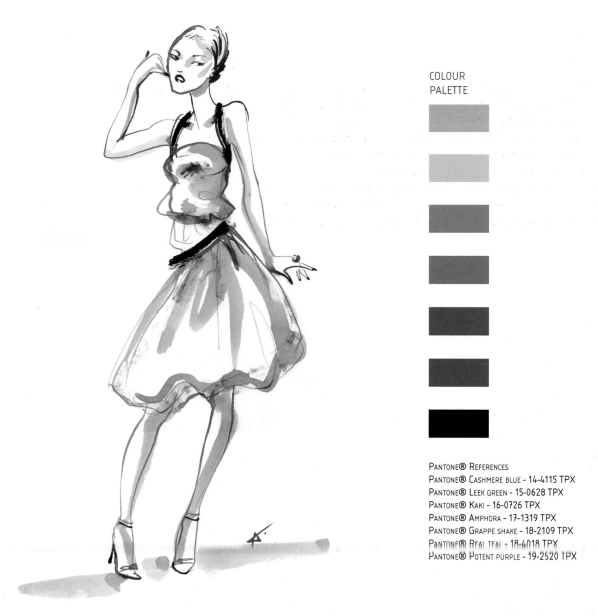

COLOUR
PALETTE

PANTONE® REFERENCES
PANTONE® CASHMERE BLUE - 14-4115 TPX
PANTONE® LEEK GREEN - 15-0628 TPX
PANTONE® KAKI - 16-0726 TPX
PANTONE® AMPHORA - 17-1319 TPX
PANTONE® GRAPPE SHAKE - 18-2109 TPX
PANTONE® REAL TEAL - 18-4018 TPX
PANTONE® POTENT PURPLE - 19-2520 TPX

The palette

To define the colours of a collection or range, it is an idea to choose an image, or photo, which is linked to the proposed theme and to extract as many colours as possible. This will then serve as the starting point for the 'palette'. The choice of the 'mood' visual is very important as the chosen colours will determine next season's trends.

Furthermore, the visuals and selected colours must correspond to the fabric of the intended garment. For example, the colour palette is much richer for printed garments and knitwear than it is for coats and suits.

The palette organises the colours into 'families' from light to dark; saturated ('pure') colours, bright, acid, fluorescent, shiny, metallic, neutral, dark, light, pastel, 'greys' etc. They can also define the shades of all the tones between two colours e.g. the shades of orange are found between yellow and magenta), colour gradation (by adding white to make lighter or, black to make darker). The shades and gradations are most often used in printing.

On this page and the following ones, we are showing two different palettes, an autumn one and a summer one. If several colour palettes are proposed for the same collection, it is essential that they are radically different in order to justify their use.

The colour way

From the palette, the designer selects the colours destined for the collection, classifying them from light to dark. This constitutes what is termed the 'colour way'. It is important that this range stays as true to the original photo as possible.

The stylist must be careful not to choose similar colours which will compete with each other. In a well-balanced range, one finds nuances of yellow, magenta and cyan, they being the three primary colours which, with the aid of white and black, recreate all the colours perceptible to the human eye.

Note that the colour ranges destined for printing are clearly broader to allow for more freedom and richness in the colouring of the motif.

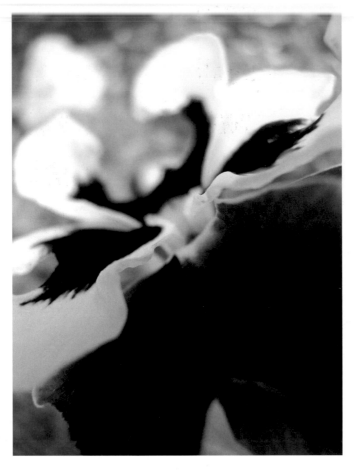

PALETTE

PANTONE® REFERENCES
PANTONE® PALE KHAKI - 15-1216 TPX
PANTONE® NATURAL - 16-1310 TPX
PANTONE® APRICOT - 15-1153 TPX
PANTONE® MULBERRY - 17-3014 TPX
PANTONE® BEETROOT PURPLE - 18-2143 TPX
PANTONE® CANYON ROSE - 17-1520 TPX
PANTONE® APRICOT BRANDY - 17-1540 TPX
PANTONE® PLUM WINE - 18-1411 TPX
PANTONE® LAGOON - 16-5418 TPX

The harmonies

From the colour range, the designer decides the colour harmonies which will be used within the collection. These can be constructed by deciding the colour balance between the colours themselves and to which proportions they are found in the different garments.

HARMONY

PALETTE

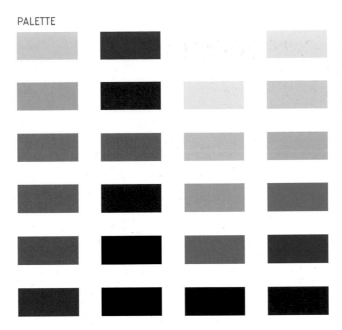

Colour Organisation

The designer can use different media to produce the palettes, colour ranges and harmonies: ink, gouache, watercolour, marker pens for the quick 'roughs' and of course, graphic software.

To avoid any eventual error of colour interpretation, colour charts exist which are specifically aimed at professional graphic, fashion and interior designers. These classify and list the nuances which correspond to a particular field (a textile colour chart, for example) thus guaranteeing a true colour reproduction.

Finally, for the ranges and harmonies, it can be interesting to use fabric samples to provide the desired colour. It is the luminosity of Lurex, the matt quality of linen, the shiny quality of silk, the depth of wool ... which aid to compile a colour range.

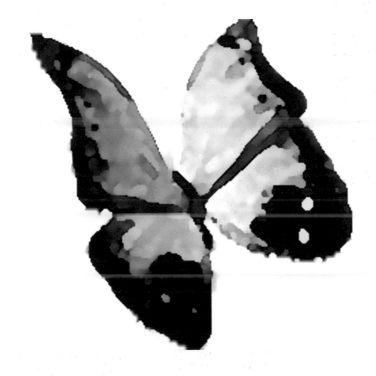

Fibres

Understanding fabrics and therefore the fibres from where they originate, is essential to the realisation of a collection. Fibres can be of natural origin (animal in the case of wool and vegetable in that of cotton, linen and hemp) or chemical (such as viscose, rayon and polyesters).

They have their own particular characteristics which determine specific applications. Linen and cotton, for example, will be more likely to be used in spring-summer collections where lightness is important whereas wool, with its thermal qualities, would be more appropriately used in autumn-winter ones. Synthetic fabrics, with their strength and heat-regulating qualities, will be destined for sportswear such as parkas and ski clothing, whereas Lycra, which is stretchy and comfortable, will be found in lingerie, dance wear and swimming costumes.

The yarns made from these fibres differ from each other depending on their diameter and type of twist. These are multiple thread assemblies which are used in a variety of ways/treatments such as sewing, lacquering, felting, bonding etc. depending on which fabric is being made.

Cloths and weaves

The weaving of yarns is carried out according to different systems, known as 'weaves' which vary depending on the fibre's origin. The three principal weaves are plain, or canvas, weave (straight weave), used for cotton poplin in shirts, twill weave (diagonal weave), which is used in the manufacture of gabardine for raincoats and trousers and finally, satin or sateen weave, derived from twill weave, which works as well with silk as it does with cotton. (It is often used for cotton moleskin in certain military style jackets.)

Knitwear and non-woven fabrics

In addition to weaving or 'yarn-dyed' fabric, there is knitwear, which consists of 'cut-and-sew' and knitted fabrics (see Chapter 1, p. 50). Industrially-knitted yarn on a roll, like cloth (called ' warp and weft') is destined for cut-and-sew garments such as soft, sweatshirt materials and jersey fabrics used in tee-shirts, dresses or trousers. Knitwear made by a system of gauges of stitch, which decrease at the sleeves and collars with ribbed trimmings on the edges and cuffs, give the finished product a 'hand-knitted' jumper feel.

Finally, there are 'non-woven' fabrics which are neither yarn-dyed nor knitted, like the felt used for the underside of suit collars and, more and more, for clothing accessories and decoration.

To illustrate these ideas, we present a selection of fabrics, by garments, corresponding to current fashions.

France remains very competitive for the manufacture of the fabrics known as 'breathable' such as poplin, silk (Lyon), embroidered fabrics, notably in lace (Calais) - as well as embellishing fabrics by washing and dyeing. Unfortunately, most of the time these fabrics are made abroad.

Suppliers of other types of fabrics are spread out over Europe. Germany specialises in felt and loden, Switzerland in fine cottons, embroidery and certain laces, Scotland in tweed and Italy produces all sorts of fabrics!

Professional fabric fairs such as Première Vision in Paris, Tissu Premier in Lilles and the Italian fairs are a 'must' for young designers. It gives them the opportunity to meet suppliers and serves as an indispensable source of information about new products and the latest innovative technologies in the textile industry.

Skirts

The fabrics are chosen in relation to the model: stretch jean material, or stretch satin, for a straight skirt and cotton poplin, or printed silk, for a petticoat.

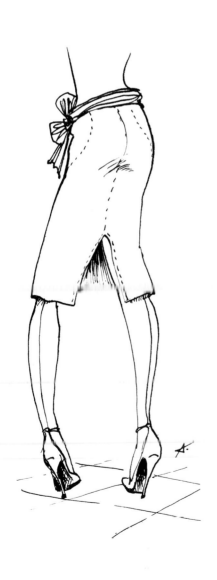

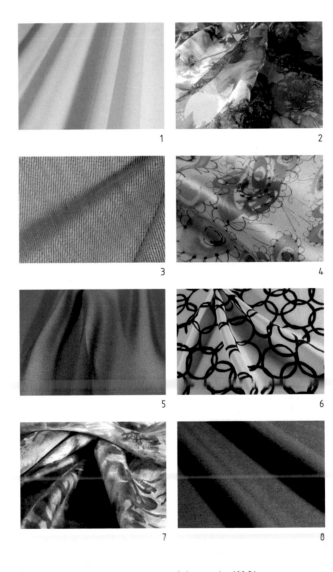

1. Jersey crêpe 100 % viscose.
2. Printed muslin crépon 100 % silk.
3. Two-coloured denim raw bicolore 100 % cotton.
4. Multi-coloured printed shantung 100 % silk..
5. Georgette 100 % polyamide.
6. Two-coloured printed Crêpe de Chine 100 % silk.
7. Satin jacquard imprimé 100 % soie.
8. Woollen crêpe 100 % wool.

Dress

The fabrics are chosen in relation to the cut and style of the
dress. Flowing jersey or voile are used for daywear with satin,
lace or taffetas for cocktail dresses or evening wear.

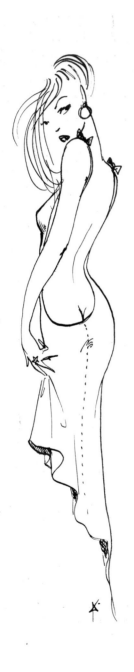

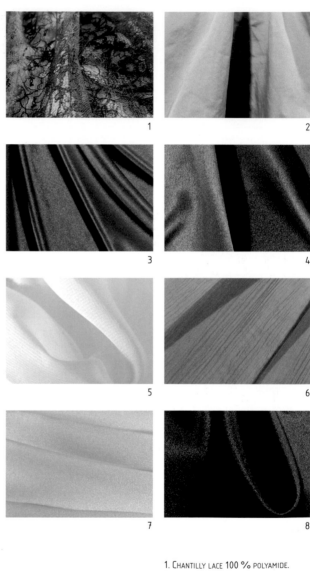

1. CHANTILLY LACE 100 % POLYAMIDE.
2. SHOT TAFFETAS 100 % SILK.
3. FLOWING JERSEY, WITH A METALLIC ASPECT, 100 % NYLON.
4. LIGHT SATIN 100 % SILK.
5. VOILE 100 % POLYESTER.
6. SHOT CHIFFON CRÉPE 100 % SILK.
7. LINGERIE SATIN 100 % SILK.
8. HEAVY SATIN-BACKED CRÊPE, (SILK + VISCOSE).

Trousers

Fashion favours jeans however, the more classic trousers are cut using masculine fabrics such as woollen poplin *fil-à-fil* or yarn on yarn (where a white thread is interwoven with a coloured one) or stripes. Street wear trousers are made from military gabardine or soft jersey.

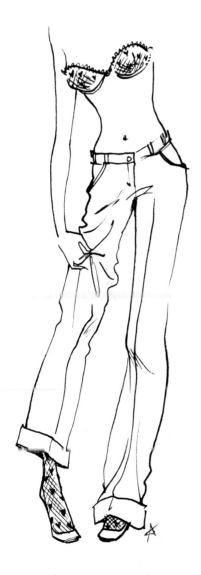

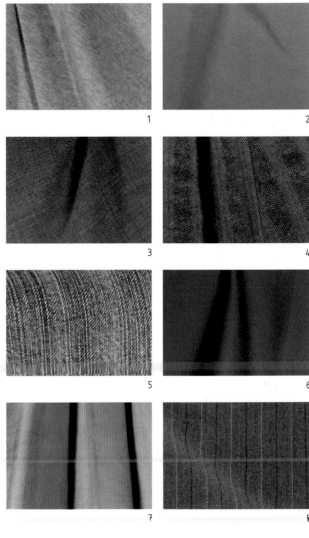

1. Soft jogging 100 % cotton.
2. Gabardine Chinos 100 % cotton.
3. Chiné or warp dyed grey double crêpe (wool + polyamide).
4. Two coloured shaded stripes (53 % paper + 47 % wool).
5. Irregular threaded vintage look jean material 100 % cotton.
6. Military style canvas cloth 100 % cotton.
7. Fine velvet corduroy 100 % cotton.
8. Double striped masculine crêpe 100 % wool.

Jacket

The fabrics most frequently used for jackets are those inspired by military wardrobes or sophisticated fabrics such as velvet or satin.

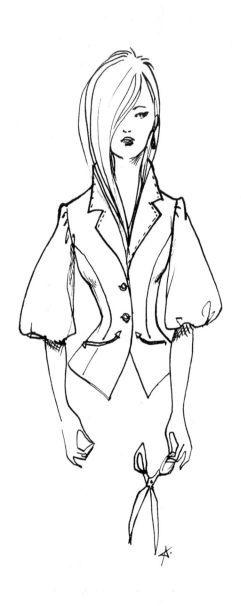

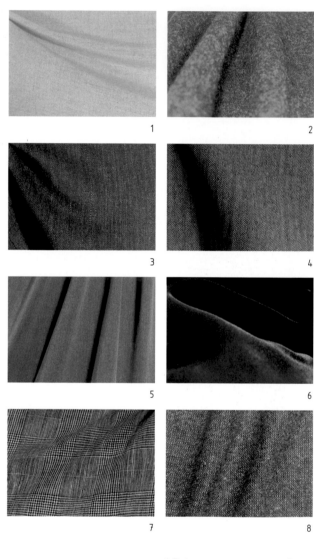

1. FIL À FIL YARN ON YARN SHANTUNG (LINEN + SILK).
2. FLANNEL 100 % WOOL.
3. MIXED CRÊPE (WOOL + POLYAMIDE).
4. SMALL HERRINGBONE WITH VINTAGE ASPECT (LINEN + COTTON).
5. CLOUDY POPLIN (COTTON + POLYAMIDE + LYCRA).
6. VINTAGE LOOK VELVET (SILK + VISCOSE).
7. PRINCE OF WALES 100 % LINEN.
8. TWEED (COTTON + WOOL + LYCRA).

Coat

Coat material is inspired by men's fabrics such as tweed or woollen cloth, or those which exude luxury and warmth, such as fur or cashmere.

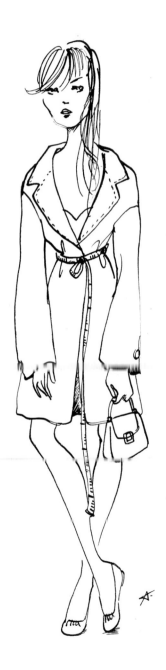

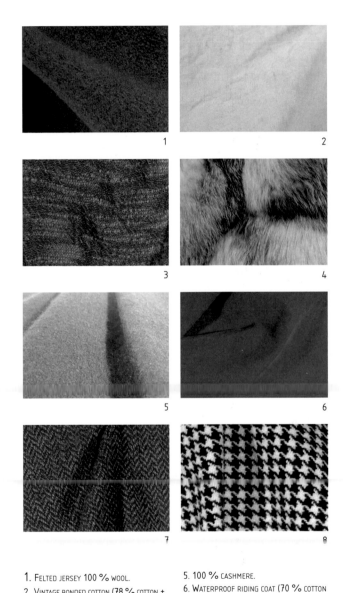

1. Felted jersey 100 % wool.
2. Vintage bonded cotton (78 % cotton + 2 % EA + 20 % PU).
3. Irregular rustic look cotton 100 % cotton.
4. Rabbit fur.
5. 100 % cashmere.
6. Waterproof riding coat (70 % cotton + 30 % polyester).
7. Harris tweed aspect chevron 100 % wool (Ireland).
8. Houndstooth check 100 % wool.

Tee-shirt

Cotton jersey is the original tee-shirt material. Nowadays, comfort and lightness are sought after, as well as sophistication. These are found in synthetically-mixed fabrics such as cotton jersey/Lycra or silk jersey/polyamide.

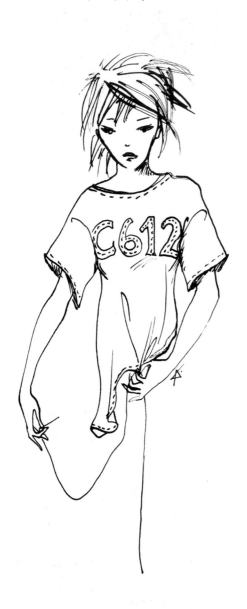

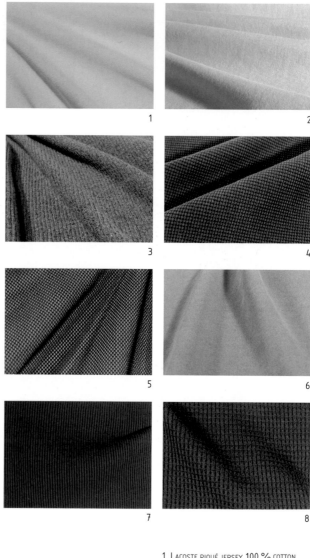

1. LACOSTE PIQUÉ JERSEY 100 % COTTON.
2. INTERLOCK JERSEY CRÊPE 100 % COTTON
3. RIBBED JERSEY (LUREX 80 % + COTTON 20 %).
4. HEAVY HONEYCOMB JERSEY 100 % COTTON.
5. FISHNET 100 % POLYAMIDE.
6. SINGLE JERSEY SIPLE (LYCRA + COTTON).
7. RIBBED JERSEY 1/1 100 % COTTON.
8. HONEYCOMB JERSEY (80 % SILK, 20 % COTTON).

Shirt/blouse

The chosen fabrics for shirts tend to be classic such as cotton poplin which are often mixed with Lycra. The preferred fabrics are light and even transparent ones like muslin and voile.

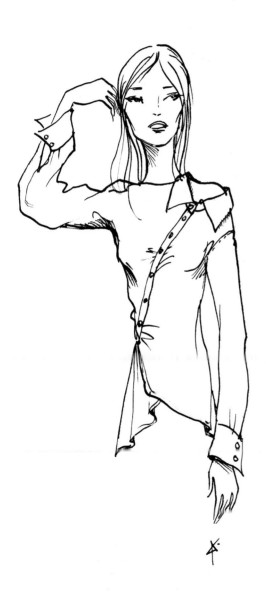

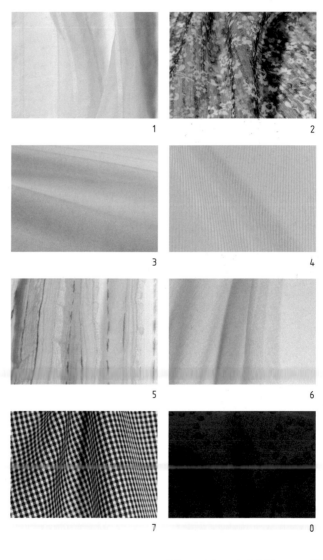

1. TRAMLINE STRIPES THREADED ONTO VOILE 100 % POLYESTER.
2. PRINTED GEORGETTE 100 % POLYESTER.
3. ORGANDY WITH GAUZE LOOK 100 % COTTON.
4. STITCHED COTTON 100 % COTTON.
5. IRREGULAR THREADED CRÊPON 100 % COTTON.
6. MUSLIN WITH IRIDESCENT LOOK 100 % POLYESTER.
7. GINGHAM SQUARED CLOTH 100 % SILK.
8. SWISS MUSLIN WITH POLKA DOTS 100 % COTTON.

What we understand by motif is the graphic interpretation of an inspiration element, used individually ('placed' motif) or in an organised composition (motif known as 'repetition' or 'repeat motif'). In the case of a repeat motif, this composition is indefinitely duplicated to cover the whole of surface area of the fabric – this is called 'printed'. One distinguishes the all-over motif such as the regular dot, for example, which is duplicated in both directions of the fabric, from the 'repeat' motif which is only reproduced in one direction as with the figurative elements of a *toile de Jouy* or with stripes. (The latter ones are known as 'Bayaderes stripes' when they are horizontal and perpendicular to the selvedge of the fabric, and 'Peking stripes' when they are vertical.)

A motif is chosen in relation to the collection's theme and will be the object of diverse developments within the range. Moreover, print can be the central focus of a range, as in the case of Louis Vuitton's line of accessories which were designed by the Japanese artist Takashi Murakami.

Several factors define the motif such as its graphics, colours, chosen background and the manufacturing techniques. The interpretation of the inspirational element can be abstract or figurative: if your image source is a flower, as in our examples, you could work along the lines of Andy Warhol's graphics which would, in turn, create a Pop Art print; for a more romantic print, a visit to the florists could aid inspiration.

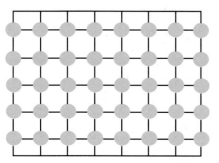

STRAIGHT REPEAT

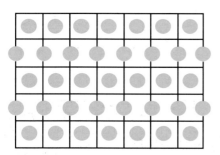

BRICK REPEAT

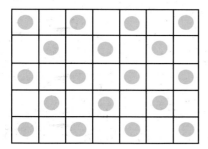

CHESSBOARD REPEAT

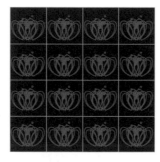

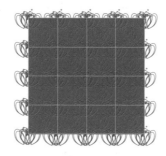

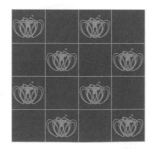

Design of textile motifs

To create a motif a scaled maquette and a sketch, showing its position on the garment, will be necessary. Maquettes are made by the textile designer, in gouache, as Sonia Delauney did for Chanel and other fashion designers, or with the aid of CAD (Computer-Aided Design) software. The technical processes are described at the end of this chapter. After digitisation, in the case of a gouache or acrylic maquette, the designs are industrially reproduced on the fabrics according to different printing techniques which are explained as follows.

To be precise a motif design, as well as a printed maquette, is termed a 'textile design'.

Several maquettes of a textile design with an all-over floral motif are presented on these two pages, accompanied by an outline showing the two types of possible organisation or 'repeat' of the motif: straight and half drop or brick repeat, the chessboard being just one variation of a straight repeat.

Note that the mock-up of an all-over

motif varies in relation to the use of the motif in the textile design (motif leans in different directions as is portrayed in the illustration on p. 77). All the variations of the motif must be taken into account before its duplication. The same is done for the number of colours used, the multiplication of which implies a different repeat.

Square-shaped scarves can use the mirror technique where duplication is done by constructing a motif in just a quarter of the piece.

Silk screenprinting

Screenprinting is the most common method of printing all-over motifs in large quantities. This is done, by the metre, on fabrics to be used as accessory lines (scarves), home products (tablecloths) and clothes (tee-shirts, blouses etc.).

In this technique, originating from traditional *savoir faire*, the motif is printed using an inked-up meshed screen within which a stencil is placed. Areas are masked off or left open depending on the pattern. The screen was originally made of silk (hence the name) stretched over a wooden frame. Today the screens are made from Terylene gauze and the frames from metal. The colours are pulled through the mesh using a squeegee using a different screen for each colour way. This 'false' four-colour printing technique gives good quality results and allows for large repeats. The recent ink-jet cylinder technique, where the colours are all injected at the same time, does not work well for large repeats and is of inferior quality.

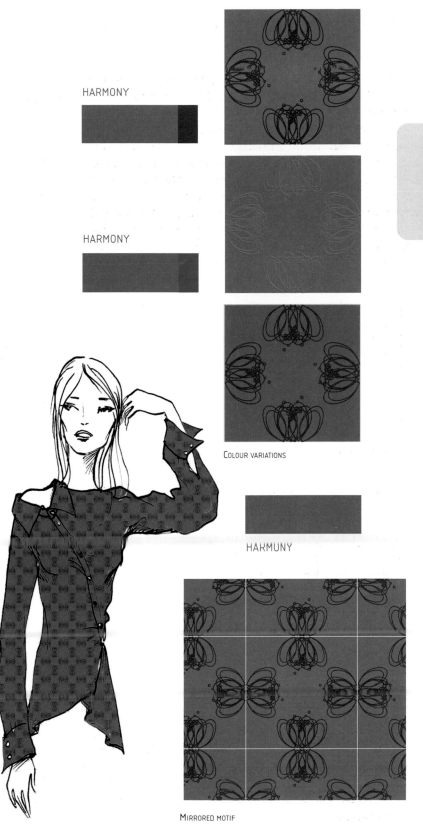

HARMONY

HARMONY

COLOUR VARIATIONS

HARMONY

MIRRORED MOTIF

The size, colour and frequency of the motif's repetition defines the different categories of printing. The Liberty print patterns, for example, are easily distinguishable with their 'carpet' of little flowers using larger ones on the wall papers; there are also 'placed' flowers and figurative ones or, contrarily, stylised and abstracted ones; those of a baroque style which use the *fleur de lys* in complex compositions; the pointillist effect of Monet's water lilies and the glimmering of Klimt's flowers – there are an infinite number of floral motifs which can be reconstructed by researching art and historical references.

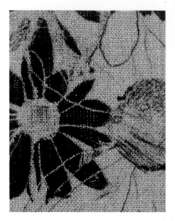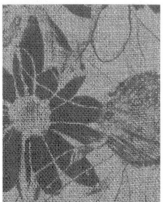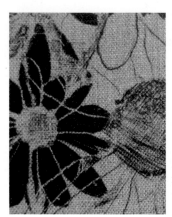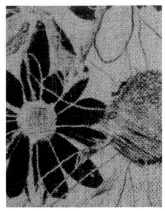

COLOUR VARIATIONS OF A FLORAL MOTIF USING SILK-SCREEN-PRINTING ON RAW LINEN.
THE COLOUR TREATMENT IS REMINISCENT OF ANDY WARHOL'S FAMOUS PRINTS.
THE OBVIOUS WEFT OF THE FABRIC ADDS TO THE TEXTILE DESIGN.

Variation of motif size

Hound's tooth check, its larger version and twill fabric squares, which have been slightly stretched diagonally, are all good examples of the effect of altering the motif size. As with these jacquard motifs, their variations make it possible to create all-over patterns.

On the next page you will see two different treatments of the same all-over floral printed motif. Used on a small scale it is reminiscent of a traditional Japanese kimono whereas, when exaggerated, it acquires a Pop Art aspect.

Choice of background fabric

The choice of background is very important as it determines the style and execution of the print and base colour, whether shiny or matt. The motifs and colours will have very different aspects according to its texture, base colour and whether it is shiny or matt.

As a general rule of thumb, white backgrounds are recommended for most prints because they enable the exact reproduction of the pattern and chosen colours. Cotton poplin, for example, offers an opaque and smooth background due to its close weave allowing for a sharp motif outline with clearly defined colours.

On the other hand a raw linen cloth, showing the natural colour of the fibre, modifies the printed colours' tones (this must be taken into account during their preparation) and will render the motif matt in appearance. Moreover, on this type of absorbent and rough cloth, it is difficult to achieve sharp definition therefore it is inadvisable to choose a very detailed motif. Although the weft can give some interesting effects.

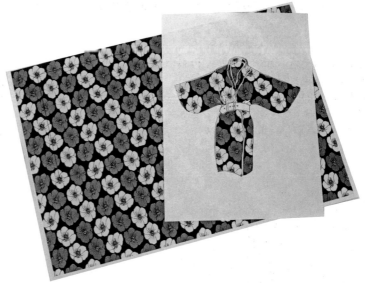

TEXTILE DESIGN WITH ALL-OVER PATTERN WITH A BRICK REPEAT. IN ORDER TO CREATE ANOTHER USE OF THIS DESIGN, THE STENCIL OF A FLAT GARMENT WAS CUT OUT AND PLACED ONTO THE PRINT. TO OBTAIN A VISIBLE RESULT – A SMALL POP ART PRINT KIMONO DRESS – IT IS NECESSARY TO MAKE A NEW MAQUETTE, DRAWN TO SCALE AND DELINEATED BY THE PENCIL MARKS, OF THE PRINT WITH MUCH LARGER MOTIFS.

In the case of a chiffon, the transparent texture of the fabric gives a diaphanous aspect to the colours which, due to refraction, become faded as the light makes them less opaque.

On these three different types of support, the printing of the same motif with the same colours will give a completely different aspect and variation of the print.

Colour combination and varieties

A colour variation can be obtained by modifying the background colour without changing that of the motif, or the reverse i.e. by changing that of the motif and not the background colour, or a combination of the two. In the case of the motif whose initial colour is red on a blue background, there are several possibilities such as: red motif on a green background, green motif on a blue background, blue motif on a green background.

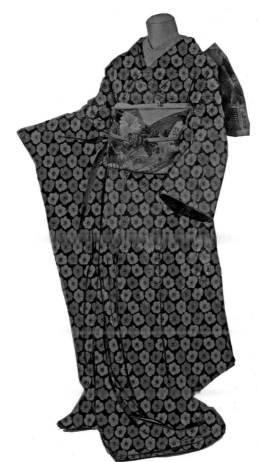

THE FINISHED RESULT OF THE SCALED MAQUETTE IS PRESENTED IN THIS KIMONO SHOWING THE COLOUR VARIATIONS USING SOMBRE TONES WHICH GIVES THE PRINT A RATHER AUSTERE LOOK.

Placed motif

When a single motif is used on a garment, it can either be applied by embroidery, patchwork, printing or transfer. The frieze pattern is a type of placed motif, running lengthwise or along the width of the fabric, thus distinguishing itself from the all-over pattern. Examples of this are when motifs embellish the bottom of a garment, such as a dress or trousers, and when jacquard patterns are used in bands on knitted jumpers. To this end, it is necessary to differentiate between the jacquard motif which is made at the same time as the weaving or the knitting of the garment, and the printed motif on a neutral background which is applied subsequently using different techniques.

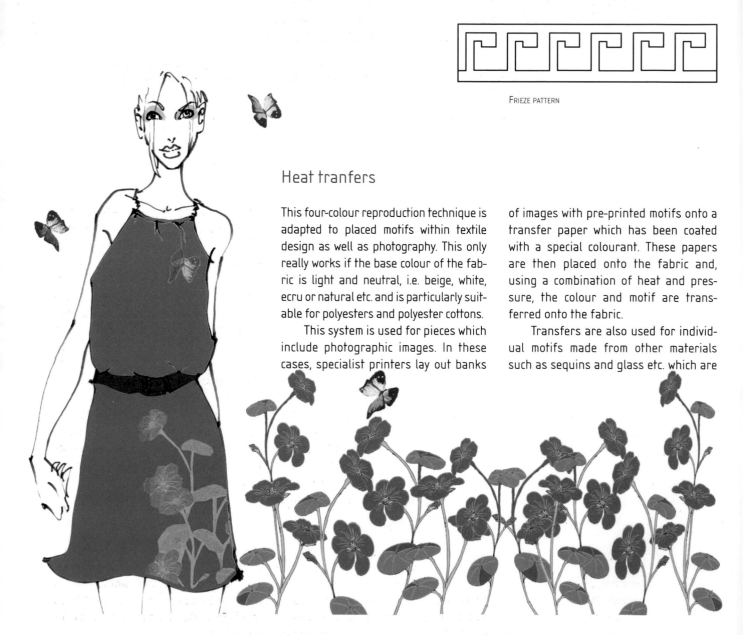

FRIEZE PATTERN

Heat tranfers

This four-colour reproduction technique is adapted to placed motifs within textile design as well as photography. This only really works if the base colour of the fabric is light and neutral, i.e. beige, white, ecru or natural etc. and is particularly suitable for polyesters and polyester cottons.

This system is used for pieces which include photographic images. In these cases, specialist printers lay out banks of images with pre-printed motifs onto a transfer paper which has been coated with a special colourant. These papers are then placed onto the fabric and, using a combination of heat and pressure, the colour and motif are transferred onto the fabric.

Transfers are also used for individual motifs made from other materials such as sequins and glass etc. which are

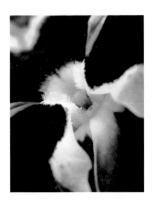

Visual inspiration.

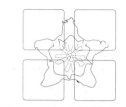

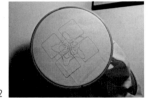

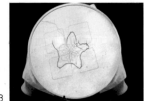

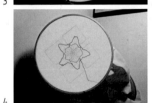

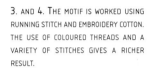

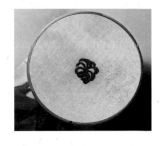

1. COMPUTER DRAWING
2. THE MOTIF IS REPRODUCED IN WASHABLE FELT PEN ONTO A COTTON CLOTH (THE FELT PEN OUTLINES WILL GRADUALLY DISAPPEAR AS THE EMBROIDERY STITCHES APPEAR). WHEN ONE WORKS WITH A NEEDLE, AS ILLUSTRATED HERE, THE CLOTH IS STRETCHED OVER A HOOP.

3. AND 4. THE MOTIF IS WORKED USING RUNNING STITCH AND EMBROIDERY COTTON. THE USE OF COLOURED THREADS AND A VARIETY OF STITCHES GIVES A RICHER RESULT.

NEEDLEPOINT EXAMPLE BEING WORKED WHERE THE OUTLINES OF THE WASHABLE FELT PEN ARE STILL NOTICEABLE. THE FLOWER IS EMBROIDERED USING A FLAT RUNNING STITCH, WITH THE EDGES FINISHED IN CHAIN STITCH.

glued directly onto the fabric using heat. The latter of which can be a satin or cotton jersey tee-shirt material. Printing onto a dark background requires a transfer technique using a white background and is described as follows.

Heat transfers on a white background

It is possible to print satisfactorily onto a dark fabric, using the heat-transfer technique, provided a white has been previously applied to the surface which is to be printed. This method is used mainly with sportswear and street wear where logos, numbers and emblems are important.

Flocking

Flocking is a printing technique which has become very popular nowadays with the growth of public interest in collective sports such as football and rugby. The relief and texture which it gives to the printed motif, as well as the contrast with the printed background, lends itself to sports and street wear such as swimsuits, tee-shirts, caps and bags whether they are knitted or made from jersey material.

The 'flock' motif, from where the technique derives its name, is most often a plain colour. The technique involves printing a glue onto the fabric and projecting minutes textile fibres onto it.

For the public, flocking is normally limited to a slogan, name or number, whereas for the professionals, the choice is much larger and comprises of floral motifs, velvet-flocked onto silk or polyester chiffons, or onto taffetas and woollen cloths.

Embroidery

There is a distinction between hand and machine embroidery. Nowadays the manual technique is applied to original placed motifs, made from thread, such as monograms. These embroideries can be more, or less, in relief according to the type of thread used i.e. cotton, silk, viscose, metallic thread etc. The degree of complexity of the motifs depends on the skill of the embroiderer who can include other materials such as ribbon, lace, pearls etc.

This type of work is normally reserved for *haute couture*, originating from top specialists in the field such as Maison Lesage.

Industrial techniques allow for the larger production of badges, logos and motifs using a variety of complex threads and colours. However, the experience and skill of a master embroiderer, with his, or her, sharpness of eye and manual precision, remain inimitable.

The embroiderer establishes a descriptive list for each embroidery indicating the method of execution, which needle or crochet, and which type of stitch and threads are to be used (even mentioning the number of strands for each thread!).

Before making a maquette of a textile design the type of motif must be considered i.e. whether it is an all-over or placed motif. For an all-over motif, you must know the size of your printing screen which, in turn, will determine that of your maquette; it must be a multiple of the latter so that the duplicated motifs will line up accordingly. A placed motif will be larger or smaller depending on its position on the garment. The type of repeat pattern must also be taken into account, i.e. straight or brick repeat and, finally, the maquette needs to be to scale.

These considerations are necessary whichever technique is employed. Our example here involves a colour preparation stage. We advise using acrylics, as opposed to gouache, because they dry quickly and result in a clean and sharp finish.

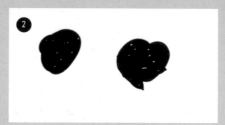

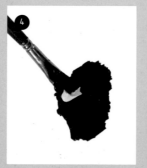

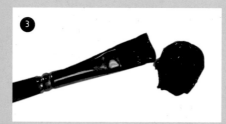

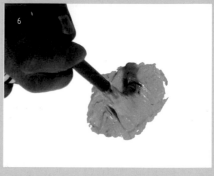

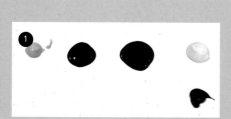

Place your colour range and visuals on the work top.

Begin by mixing the darkest colour working towards the lightest, like here mix the blue and the red together to produce violet, and then add the white to lighten the colour, or add the black to darken it.

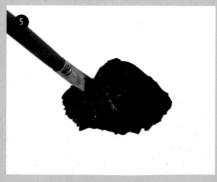

Dip the colour into a strip of paper and compare it with your colour reference chart. As gouache tends to lighten on drying, your colour must therefore be a tone, slightly darker, than your colour reference.

Create your own colours by using the three primary colours: magenta, yellow and cyan, then white and black. Commercial intermediary colours, which are the result of mixes whose proportions vary depending on the manufacturer, can in fact prevent the desired colour being obtained.

NB: To benefit from the most neutral light, work in the daylight in front of a north-facing window when using colours.

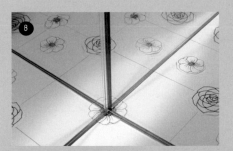

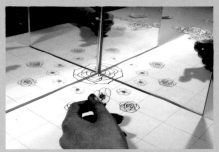

To make a square piece, such as a scarf, you can use the mirror system, which consists of placing your maquette opposite two mirrors which have been placed at 90° to each other. This allows you to work on a quarter of the design whilst visualising the whole.

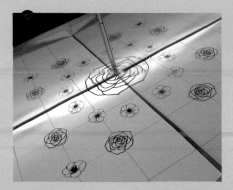

The design of a centred motif is then created, as with this rose and its mirror reflection.

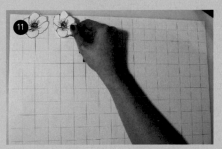

The drawing of the motif can be done by hand or by using CAD (Computer-Aided Design) software. If, like here, you work by hand, use a medium hard HB pencil to trace sharp outlines. Once the motif has been finalised, make several photocopies enlarged to the desired size (according to the envisaged textile design) with a sufficient number of copies to make your design combination.

Trace a grid in pencil on to either millimetre graph paper, tracing paper or use a computer. Place the motif on to the grid in relation to the chosen repeat (straight or brick).

So that the motif sits comfortably in the space, you can play with either the size of the motif or that of the grid. A small motif which has been placed onto a large grid will look lost, whilst too large a motif placed onto a tight grid will look too busy. To make a successful textile design the ideal situation is to balance the full areas with the spaces.

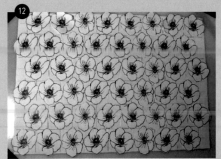

The placing of the motif is finished. Fix your motif with glue or double-sided masking tape onto the grid before placing the work onto a light box. Cover it with tracing paper and trace off the motifs' outlines using a light pencil line. This will give you a design which is ready to be coloured in.

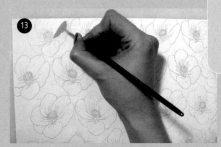

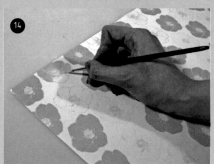

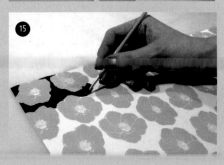

Apply your colours onto the maquette placing them next to each other without overlapping them. Even with acrylic, overlapping is not advisable as it will alter the opacity, tonality and luminosity of the colours. It is for this reason why the background must be white. With gouache, superimposing is totally inadvisable as the colours will mix together.

These step by step instructions are for a Windows computer, however, if using an Apple Mac one, the Apple key replaces the Ctrl key. Here we describe the stages needed for an all-over motif using, initially, a mirror pattern then a straight or brick repeat.

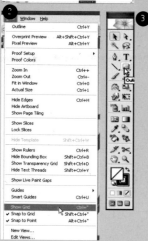

In Illustrator open the file of the motif, which is to be duplicated, and display the grid so that the motif can be correctly positioned. Then select the motif with all its corresponding elements. By using the Selection tool, trace a rectangle around the entire motif. Group these elements together using the Group command in the Object menu (or Ctrl +G). In the Tool palette, select the rectangular icon. Click on the work space and slide the mouse, holding the button down, whilst pressing the Maj key (or Shift) to obtain a square.

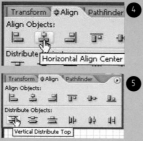

Select the square and the motif then, with the aid of the Align palette (menu Window – Align) place the motif at top of the square centring it widthways using the horizontally-centred Align icon and Distribute icon.

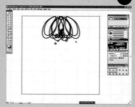

To create a single object, select the square and motif again and combine them by simultaneously pressing the Ctrl + G keys.

To duplicate them, select this set, click and slide it, whilst simultaneously pressing the Alt (or Ctrl + V) key. Repeat this operation to obtain 4 sets. Select the first set and pivot it 90° (menu Object – Transform – Rotate). Select the second set and pivot it 180°. Select the third set and, this time, pivot it 270°. The fourth set stays in the same place. This will give you the result in Fig. 7.

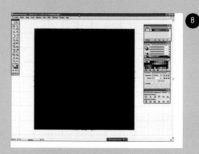

Select the 4 sets. In the Align window, select the following options: centrally – vertical Align and centrally- horizontal Align. This will give you the result in Fig. 8.
Select the 4 sets again and select the Ungroup command in the Object menu in order to divide them into groups. Then select 3 of the 4 squares and delete them using the Delete key so that only the outline of the initial square is visible.

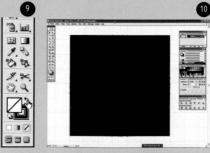

Select the square and begin by inverting the properties of the outline and fill-in by clicking on the small black arrow in the Tool palette. The colour properties are symbolised by two squares, one representing the line, the other the fill-in. The red diagonal line which appears in the colour square indicates that, for the moment, no colour has been selected. To add a background colour, double-click on the fill-in key. A colour selector appears. Choose the desired colour and click OK. You now have set up the base motif.

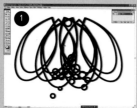

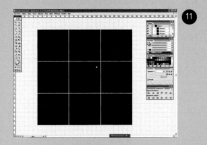

Select the set and press the Shift and G keys simultaneously to create a single object. Select this object and duplicate it until you obtain 9 of them. Using the grid, position them in such a way that a new square is created containing 9 objects. The finished motif is created.

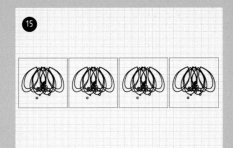

Select the object, click on it and slide it to the edge whilst simultaneously pressing the Maj (Shift) key. This will position it in the same line as the previous one. Then press the Alt key to copy it. When the mouse is released, the object will be repositioned and copied at the same time. Select the 4 successive objects and slide them in a way to line up at regular intervals on the grid.

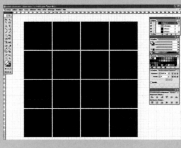

Divide the 16 objects by selecting them and pressing simultaneously on the Ctrl, Shift and G keys (or select Ungroup in the Object menu.) Select the squares and give them a background colour as previously explained on the opposite page in Fig. 9. The maquette of a straight repeat pattern for an all-over motif is now finished.

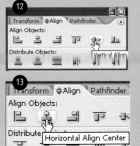

To make this motif redo the stages 1 to 3 followed by mirroring the motif. Once you have made your square, centre the motif within it.

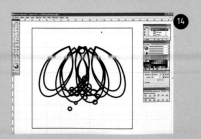

To do this, select the square and the motif using the Align palette. Select the square and the motif again and re-group them using the Ctrl and G keys.

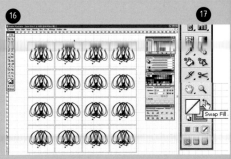

Select the set of 4 objects and slide them whilst simultaneously pressing on the Alt key (this will duplicate them) and the Maj or (Shift) key (this will align the two rows) as before.
Repeat the operation to obtain 4 lines of 4 objects, then using the grid, place them at regular intervals to create a new square containing 16 objects.

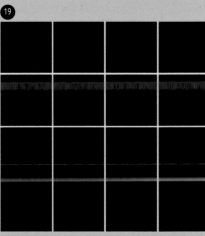

It is possible to experiment with other repeat patterns such as chess board or brick repeat. To achieve a chess board pattern as seen here, just select the elements to be removed and delete them by pressing the Delete key on the keyboard. To achieve a brick repeat pattern, select the elements of one row and displace them either using the mouse or the arrows on the keyboard as well as pressing the Maj (Shift) key to keep the alignment.

The somewhat overused term concept does, however, evoke a precise notion. It is the representation, according to the 'eyes of the spirit' of a form, an idea or a sensation. Coupled with intuition, it is the starting point for the creative process. ' Intuition without concept is blind and concept without intuition is empty.' We owe this affirmation to the German philosopher Emmanuel Kant (1724–1804) whose writings are essential reading for anybody concerned with aesthetics and is known, most notably perhaps for his work *Observations* on the sentiments of beauty and the sublime. This quotation can be applied to all the domains of art and thinking, and consequently to the fashion world and its creative process.

Thus, concept is upstream of 'conception' as we understand it in the fashion milieu (in the 'elaboration' sense) which is the result as manufacture is the last stage of the creation of a garment.

Although there are numerous methods of creation, as we show here, used equally in architecture and the plastic arts, they will all be founded on the definition of a concept or creation principle. The general idea of the collection and its theme, conform to the idea, image and concept which originate from the creator, or, designer.

In the fashion world, the concept is the synthesis, as Emmanuel Kant suggests, for all the arts in general. That is why, in this book, the Concept chapter comes after Colours and Fabrics but before Visual Presentation. A theme, or an image, evokes certain colours and textures which, in turn, correspond to precise fabrics and accessories. For example, the idea 'British Amazon' could infer horse-riding, therefore leather and tweed with knee-high boots. A line originating from this concept could include jodhpurs (as in Hitchcock's film *Marnie*) but also elegant dresses for women who ride side-saddle (as with Scarlett O'Hara in *Gone with the Wind*). These two types of women are united by the same concept.

Without a solid concept, no visual representation can be properly understood. The concept is one of the conditions of a good communication of ideas and information between the designer and the merchandiser, but also between themselves and their numerous collaborators. From this point of view, looking at the fashion metiers from every angle, concept is, in itself, a strategy.

According to the definition given in the dictionary, strategy is 'the art of advancing an army onto a theatre of operations up to the point where it comes in contact with the enemy'. This definition can equally suit advertising where one speaks of advertising 'campaigns' using the analogy of military campaigns, although in this case, the conquest is one of an offensive by seduction! Replacing the term 'army' by 'team or design studio', the term 'enemy' by 'public' (for it is the public who needs to be conquered by pleasing or surprising, as well as, anticipating its expectations), a creative strategy can be put in place for a brand or fashion house. For example, the different stages of the conceptual approach, combination of ideas, reflections and intuitive actions can be compared to that of a military operation. In the context of a collection's conception, this will consist of transforming images, sources of inspiration, into fabrics, colours, forms and styles in order to create a complete universe. Still likening this to a military exercise, the manoeuvres will use every means possible to design and develop the brand.

In this chapter we break the concept down into two parts, that of the development of the concept and, that of the drawing up of the collection, the first concentrates on the conceptual creative process whilst the second deals with the research of shapes and lines, through sketches and 3D, and the tools necessary for this.

Concept also encompasses the previously presented product. The variations in the complete product line ranges, in view of satisfying and anticipating the client's demand, is in fact planned in the concept and, in turn, it is these proposed products which define the brand's image. However, the concept can be derived from a particular garment and its feel – loose (dress, blouse), fitted (jacket, suit), structured or unstructured. In every case, the process is done in stages, continually redefining the product in relation to its target – the client.

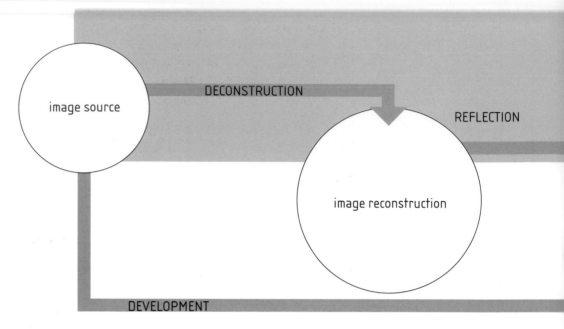

THIS DIAGRAM SHOWS THE OPERATIONAL DEVELOPMENT OF THE CONCEPT.

Stage 1

This is the research phase. The first step is to gather together the inspirational elements needed. In the chosen example, after having analysed three 'elements', a flower (the pansy), a gladiator's peplum and his armour, we have loosely interpreted them to see how they might overlap. The image source is then deconstructed into abstract representations of the three constituent elements.

Stage 2

The second stage is to analyse the elements in their initial state: in our example we have picked up on the crumpled aspect of the flower, with its transparent petals and curved outline. From the pep-lum, we have taken the blousy and feminine aspects found in the folds and from the gladiator, we have derived strength and rigour from the belt. The designer confronts these characteristics at the concept stage then organises them choosing the theme which will translate his ideas the best. This stage defines the objectives and the direction that the whole studio will take for the season.

The designer then develops his themes using original details to give an identity to his creations such as in our example i.e. large folds, pleats, drapes, blousy and crumpled look, binding etc.

He or she defines the silhouettes by researching shapes (in this case, light-weight garments: blousy dresses, puff ball skirts and superimposing volume and fabrics), creating the colour palette (here: bold and neutrals) and selecting the fab-rics (here: light floating ones: crêpe, satin worked into gathered details, voiles etc.).

Stage 3

The third stage is the synthesis of this work process, the variation of the collec-tion i.e. deciding on which product (in this case, a dress and tunic) and the cre-ation of its environment: boutiques, the type of event, organisation of commer-cial showrooms, choice of models, their hairstyles, make-up, choice of photogra-pher and setting etc.

The entire ensemble of these ele-ments will affirm the brand's identity.

STUDIES

CONTROLS
- organisation
- commercial viability
- level of innovation
- conveying of message
- originality

ASSIMILATION

GARMENTS
- photos
- illustrations
- beauty
- computer graphics
- etc.

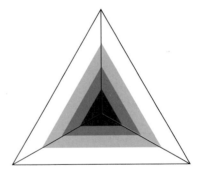

commerciability

coherence
image control

innovation
creativity

Creation and commercialisation

The prism above indicates the three points of development for the concept: creation, image and marketing and the balance which must be established between them in order to commercialise an innovative product which has its own identity.

However, one can orientate a collection in relation to the results of the preceding ones and the public's response. For example, if the design and image had been well-received last season, the following season could be directed towards a more commercial approach.

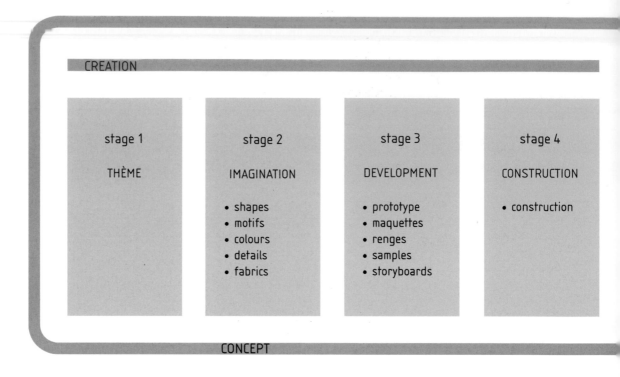

The concept

The concept is the basis of the work as it defines the direction of a collection. It determines the transformation and fusion of the various inspirational materials derived from historical, ethnological, sociological sources, or drawn from nature. The example found in the following pages uses a cocoon as the concept. It is inspired by the same visuals as those used for the theme, i.e. the flower, the peplum and gladiator armour. However, this does not always have to be the case.

Stage 1 – Theme

The theme evolves with the seasons. There can be one, or several, in a collection and it is directly influenced by the concept. For example, the original concept of Issey

Miyake's pleats was derived from architecture. These have been reinterpreted in successive collections using different themes with acid and bright colours.

Paco Rabanne's concept is 'space' which is illustrated by using non-textile materials such as metal derived from the technology world. As previously mentioned the theme we have chosen is that of a flower associated with a peplum and gladiator armour.

Stage 2 – Conception and research

The theme is declined in sub-themes, or variations, which allow shapes, colours, motifs, details and fabrics to be imagined. Each sub-theme is the original

starting point of the general idea of a theme. The first sub-theme in our example is that of 'Ode to a Rose' with ample, supple and fluid volumes in bright colours. The second is 'The Valkyries' strapped up with wide belts in more neutral tones and the third is 'The Romantic Warrior' which unifies the whole idea and illustrates the concept of 'cocoon' by its shapes.

Stage 3 – Development

This is the developmental stage of the preceding research. After researching the shapes of the products, the *toiliste, or pattern cutter, submits a prototype sample to the designer (see Chapter 5, p. 140 onwards). The textile designer cre-

* this French term for 'pattern cutter' is in general usage

```
┌─────────────────────────────
│  ┌──────────────────
│  │  IMAGE
│  │
│  │  ┌────────────
│  │  │
│  │  │  stage 5
│  │  │
│  │  │  PRESENTATION
│  │  │
│  │  │  • photographis
│  │  │  • illustrations
│  │  │  • animations
│  │  │  • visuals
│  │  │  • sounds/music
```

INFORMATION/KNOWLEDGE
- history
- folklore
- arts
- sociology
- nature...

THIS DIAGRAM ILLUSTRATES ALL THE PROCESSES REQUIRED
TO PRODUCE A COLLECTION FROM THE GIVEN CONCEPT, ITS
CONCEPTUAL STAGES THROUGH TO ITS PRESENTATION.

ates the textile design maquettes (see Chapter 3, pp. 74-83). The designer then chooses his colour range (see Chapter 3, pp. 62-5). The samples are then made up by the pattern cutter. Finally, the person in charge of fabrics makes a selection according to the garments which are to be produced.

Stage 4 - Collection plan

This fourth stage is the gathering together of all the elements obtained in Stage 3 to produce the collection. The products are fitted into the collection plan (see Chapter 1, pp. 58-9). The merchandiser plans the season and imposes the look, the necessary accessories and brand onto the designers.

Stage 5 - Promotion

The promotional phase is initiated right at the beginning of the collection's conception. The artistic director is the principal player in this. He decides the characteristics of the presentation (see Chapter 6) destined for the press and clients and directs the entire team.

He chooses the photographers, directors and PR agencies so as to create a publicity image, and the press packs aimed at the media i.e. magazines, television and advertising.

He will also instruct an illustrator to draw the season's silhouettes and present them in a press pack for fashion editors, photo-stylists from the media and film or music companies in

order to attract magazine editorial, television and film appearances.

Eventually, he will ask an animator to produce special effects destined for the brand's website for the presentation or for the boutiques. Finally, he will instruct a music researcher to choose the soundtrack music for the fashion show, which can eventually be used in the boutiques and showrooms.

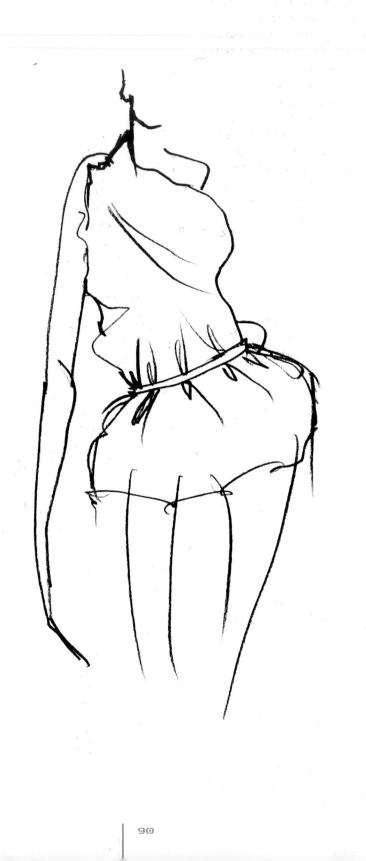

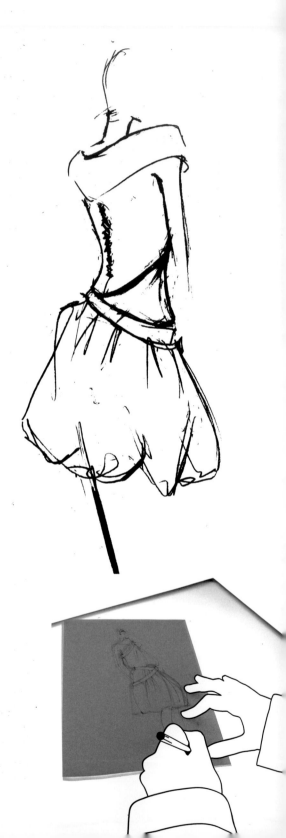

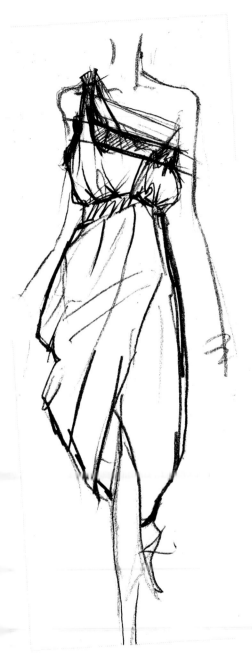

Inspired by the unity of the research surrounding the flower, the designer develops the idea further using a series of sketches corresponding to its shapes and volume referring to the fabric selection made for the season.

Traditionally, the flower evokes femininity, the same as the dress is perceived as the archetypal garment of femininity. These simple associations are at the origin of the example that we show here. The historical theme of antiquity and the peplum relate to the flower with its drapes, overlays of fabric, deep folds and pleats, transparent areas which contrast with opaque ones and with its tonal nuances. The belt of the gladiator's armour, by its crude aspect, balances the product by reinforcing the lines, tempering and directing them. The coming together of all these inspirational elements as a unit determines the silhouettes making for ample and voluminous shapes.

The flower is interpreted in a very graphic style corresponding to the general design of the project. Whilst sketching, the designer must keep in mind this inspirational unit as he creates his collection without venturing too far away from it. The silhouettes are drawn up, balancing and harmonising volume and lengths, as the collection starts to take shape.

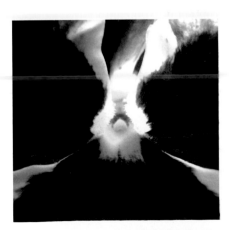

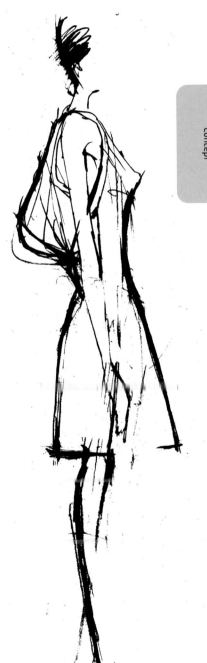

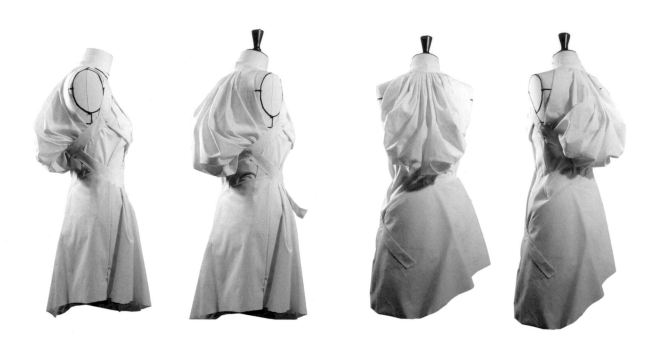

Running parallel to the sketches, the designer uses a tailor's dummy, also known as a dress form, to imagine his/her idea in three dimensions. The papier maché dummy or mannequin provides two essential reference points: the vertical axis which is placed in the centre front or of the dummy or grain line and the horizontal axis, perpendicular to the first, which is fixed at the waist.

The fall of the fabric

Shape research consists of understanding the fall of a fabric on a dummy with the help of the reference points. The fabric itself has a vertical direction known as a length, known as the lengthwise/straight grain line of the fabric, parallel to the selvedge. The length varies depending on the chosen garment whereas the width of the roll is fixed (for example, at 90 to 110 cm for silk and 140 cm plus for cotton and wool etc.) The lines traced widthways, which are perpendicular to the grain line, are called the crosswise grains. All of which give a balance to the garment.

The bias is the diagonal of the fabric (45° to the selvedge and the cross grain) (see Chapter 6, p. 151). When fabric is cut on the bias, it allows for more gracious shapes and a more subtle fabric fall. This particular technique was used a lot in the 1930s when making drapes and pleats.

Draping the fabric

One can play with the grain and direction of the fabric. By using a series of pivoting and sliding systems the designer, or *toiliste*, can reduce the volume of the drapes using tucks, pleats and gathers in the narrow areas of the body, such as the waist.

The same process can be used to exaggerate the volume and deform the silhouette. The result of this draping is known as the *toile*. This is a trial garment, made from calico or muslin, used to test pattern and fit and which can be adjusted before making the pattern (see the section regarding 'draping' in Chapter 5, pp. 150-7).

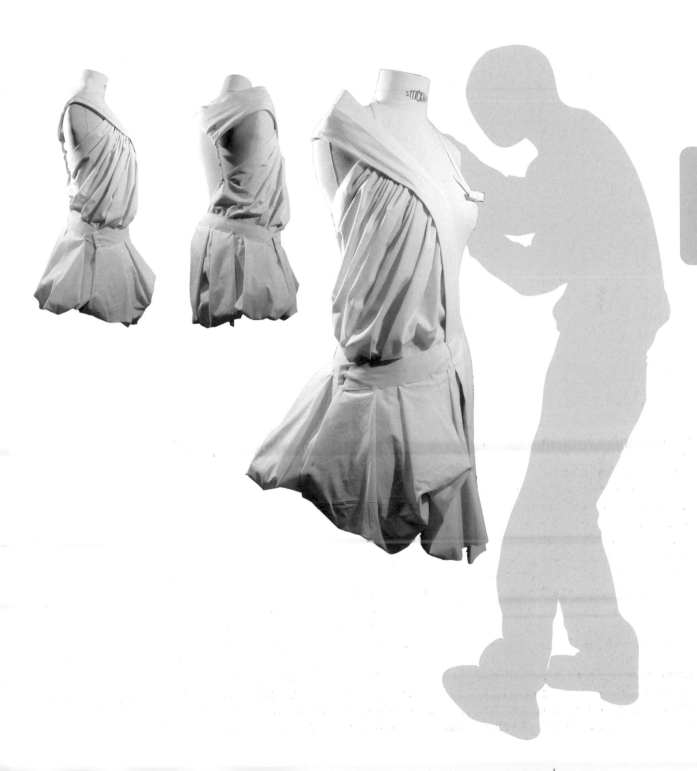

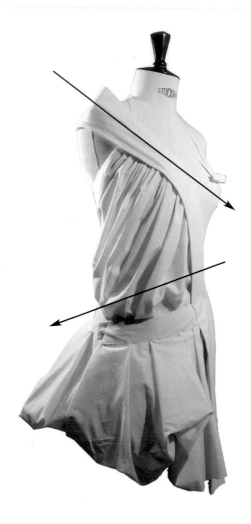

When working with asymmetrical shapes, it is advisable to visualise guidelines in order to harmonise the volumes and balance the whole. The eye naturally perceives balance and imbalance. Two diagonal lines following the same direction will be interpreted by our eye as falling. To re-establish symmetry, a line in the opposite direction will give the effect of balancing the garment.

In order to understand the notion of symmetry in fashion terms, imagine a series of match boxes piled up on top of one another to form a vertical column. If you open one of the drawers, the building will become unbalanced and fall down. On the other hand, if you simultaneously push two of the drawers in opposing directions, it will remain balanced.

The human form follows the same law of weightlessness. When we start to move our legs, the pelvis becomes lopsided, making the spinal column move sideways. Simultaneously, the shoulder axis counteracts this imbalance by leaning in the opposite direction to that of the pelvis axis. Dance, in fact, is the art of mastering the body by balancing these movements in a sequence of harmonising poses. In the fashion world, asymmetric creations require an understanding of symmetry and the balance of volumes in the right proportions.

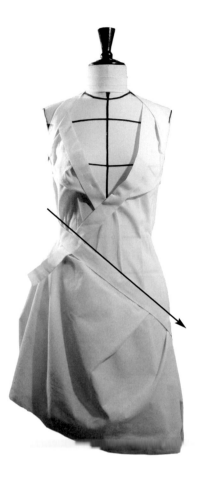

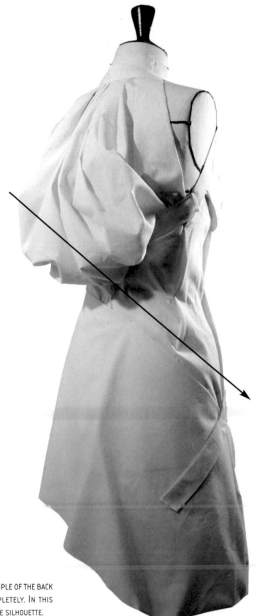

THE VOLUME OF THE BASE GIVES THE IMPRESSION OF AN OVER-
SIZED SKIRT WHICH CAN, IN THIS EXAMPLE, BE ALLOWED AS IT SITS
NATURALLY ON A SIMPLE TUNIC: A HAPPY ACCIDENT.

AN OVER-EXAGGERATED VOLUME, AS IN THIS EXAMPLE OF THE BACK
OF THIS DRESS, DEFORMS THE BODY LINE COMPLETELY. IN THIS
CASE IT IS ADVISABLE TO REDUCE THE REST OF THE SILHOUETTE.

Valkyrie theme

Colour Way

Colour Way

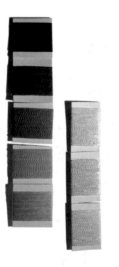

FABRICS

Iseult

Wide dress held by shoulder strap, billowing at the waist with attached 'falling' belts. Hidden side fastening.

The fashion illustration is different to that of the silhouette (see Chapter 1, pp. 32-5 and Chapter 5, p.149). The silhouette shows the volume, shapes and lengths of the collection whereas the illustration shows the products or garments. The illustration is integrated into the conceptual process as a logical progression after the stages of shape research, sketch and three-dimensional work on the mannequin. It corresponds to a maturing stage of the idea for the collection.

The fashion illustration is the result of great consideration and cannot be reduced to a stereotypical drawing. It must, therefore, have its own individual identity depicting an aspect of the world conceived by the designer. Even badly executed, an illustration which has a strong identity will be far more interesting than the calibrated and well-proportioned drawings found in certain rigid sketches! Nevertheless, it is very important to understand the proportions of the human body before trying to exaggerate them.

COSIMA

SLIGHTLY FLARED STRAP DRESS WITH AN INVERTED PLEAT IN THE FRONT AND ASYMMETRIC BIAS CUT YOKE ON THE CHEST. SKIRT WITH INLAID BELTS AND FLARED HEMLINE. HIDDEN FASTENING IN THE CENTRE OF THE BACK.

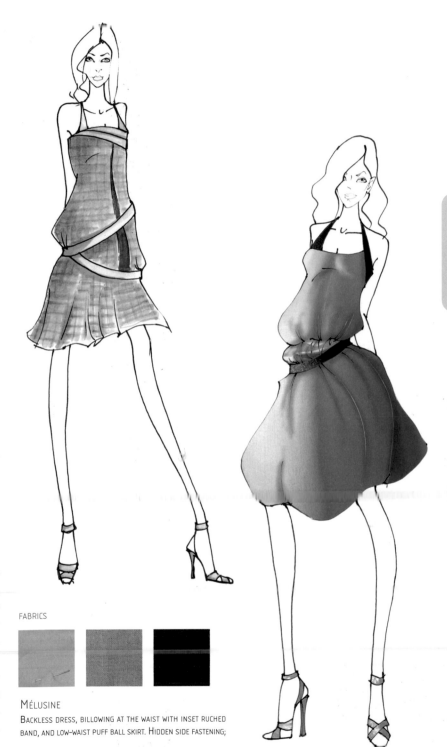

Characteristics

The modeller (the person who makes the *toile* of the garment) uses the* illustration as a model for the proposed product. The illustration serves as a method of communication between the designer and the modeller. It carries a name (or number) and is accompanied with a legend describing the garment. It is then presented with the corresponding fabric samples or swatches.

The choice of technique used, i.e. type of drawing tool, is generally left to the designer according to the product. For example, the fabric for a soft jumper could be expressed by using pastels whereas that of a gabardine raincoat would require a sharper line, possibly using a felt pen. The style of graphics can be fixed by a company in its method plan.

It is not necessary to add colour to the illustration immediately as the colours could be altered if the materials chosen for the prototype are not suitable.

FABRICS

MÉLUSINE

BACKLESS DRESS, BILLOWING AT THE WAIST WITH INSET RUCHED BAND, AND LOW-WAIST PUFF BALL SKIRT. HIDDEN SIDE FASTENING;

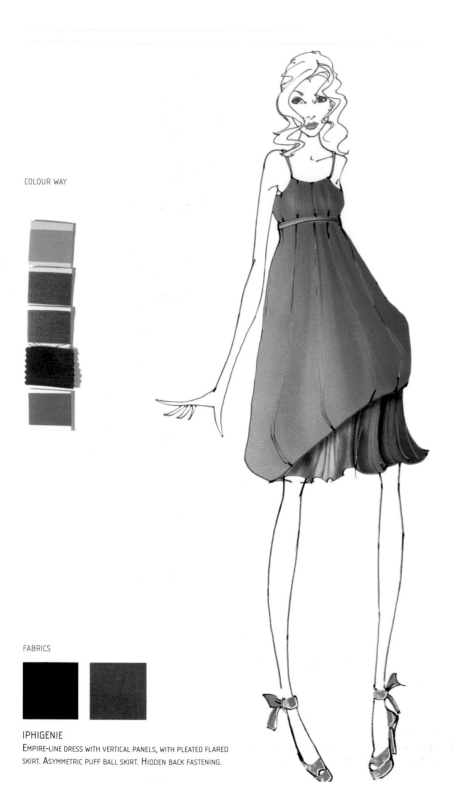

COLOUR WAY

FABRICS

IPHIGENIE
EMPIRE-LINE DRESS WITH VERTICAL PANELS, WITH PLEATED FLARED
SKIRT. ASYMMETRIC PUFF BALL SKIRT. HIDDEN BACK FASTENING.

Graphic standards

The line of the illustration is detailed and precise. Every element of the garment must be easy to understand such as the front including all the pieces which it consists of, i.e. the side, sleeves, neckline, pleats, folds, yokes, cuffs etc. Even the seams are detailed showing the precise manner in which they are to be assembled such as flat, lapped and top-stitched on one or another.

Romantic warrior theme

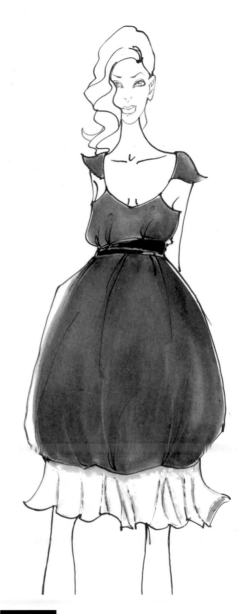

If the lines in the product are symmetrical, they will need to be reproduced as true to the drawing as possible. For example, if the angle of a neckline or collar (which is normally the symmetrical part) is not represented as symmetrical in the illustration, instead it is leaning left or right, the *toilliste* in turn will make an error. It is therefore extremely important that the illustration is as true to the idea as possible to avoid any erroneous interpretations concerning volumes, lengths or details as this can hold up the production of a collection, as well as cause bad feeling within the team.

To facilitate the understanding of a drawing in the studio, it is advisable to leave the illustration in black and white. This also allows it to be scanned after which the designer can use the computer to add fabric effects and render it in original and explicit colours. The different techniques of achieving this are explained on the following pages.

FABRICS

EUPHROSYNE
PUFF BALL COCKTAIL DRESS WITH FANCY STRAPS AND RIBBON WAISTBAND ON A PLEATED FLARED SKIRT. HIDDEN BACK FASTENING.

Colour rendering with a felt pen

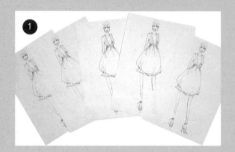

Photocopy the illustration several times so that a number of different fabric effects and colour harmonies can be tested; this way if a mistake is made there is no need to return to the original drawing.

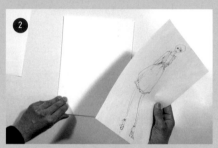

Position the illustration onto a block of rough paper to protect the table. This also allows the ink to be absorbed and avoids it 'bleeding' outside the outline of the illustration.

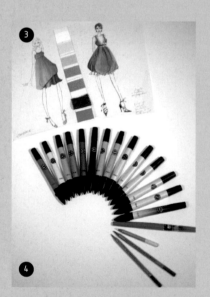

Choose a selection of felt pens which correspond to the proposed colour range. It is best to use lighter tones first then add contrasting ones later.

Watercolour crayons can also be used to emphasise the colours and accentuate the fabric effects.

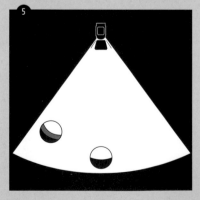

For a more contrasting look, imagine a lateral light source, coming from either, the left, or the right of the illustration, depending on the volumes which are to be accentuated. An area of shadow and light is then achieved.

Felt or marker pens are basic tools for a designer as they allow rough sketches to be colour-rendered quickly. They can be used for the final presentation (fashion plates) in conjunction with other media such as coloured crayons, paintbrushes and pen and ink etc. Although simple, the felt pen can give a certain high quality to the work.

They exist in a wide range of colours and by mixing different ones together nuances can be obtained. Felt pen manufacturers supply neutral tones (Pantones R Gray Cool and Gray Warm) for monochrome drawings which are used to accentuate shadows. The markers are also equipped with interchangeable nibs in various shapes, i.e. wide, fine, round, square, angled, rigid and flexible – all of which offer a variety and precision of line.

The nibs are made from felt or fibre. The felt ones, being more resistant, are used for a quick colour application and flat colour rendering, whereas the fibre ones tend to be used for more detailed work.

Specific papers, such as layout paper, are compatible with marker inks as they do not allow the ink to come through nor 'bleed' outside the outline of the illustration.

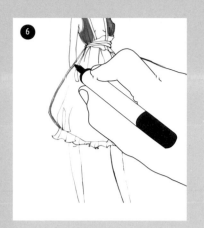

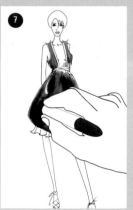

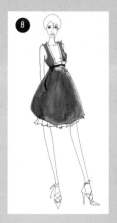

Fill in the coloured areas of the dress taking care not to go over the outline of the illustration.

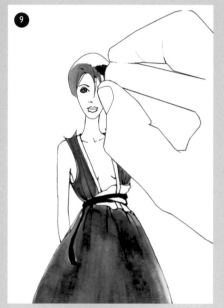

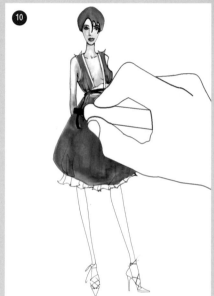

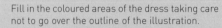

Use different coloured pens for the hair tones. For the face use the Pantone Blender-T and mix it with a skin tone one so as to give it a slight shadowing and texture. Then apply the make-up using watercolour crayons which will give it a look of transparency, similar to cosmetics.

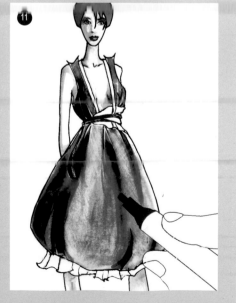

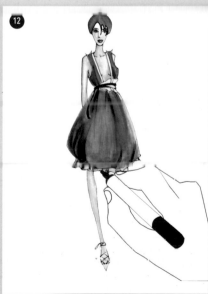

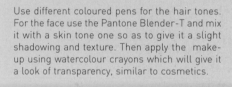

Colour in the shaded areas. In the case of a thick fabric, accentuate the shadows with opaque colours; if, however, it is sheer, use transparent colours to enhance the idea of luminosity.

To accentuate shadows, apply several layers of marker ink, allowing it to dry between each layer and, for a particularly contrasting effect, use the complementary colour.

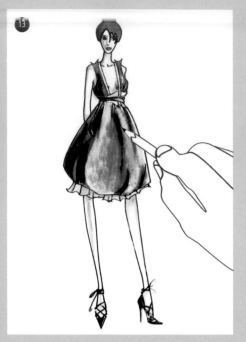

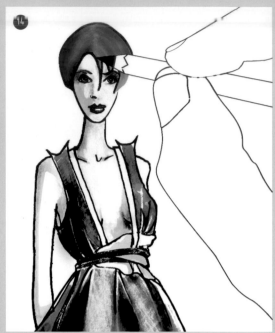

> To represent gold, silver and lame, add white dots and stars.

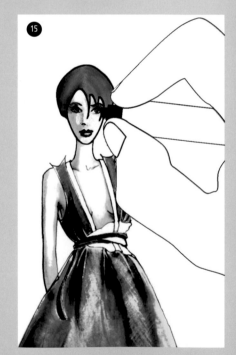

Use watercolour crayons to emphasise the highlights of a fabric – white for light areas and sombre colours for the folds etc.

Use the same technique for the hair. The combination of marker pen and watercolour crayons give a more interesting effect than if used singularly.

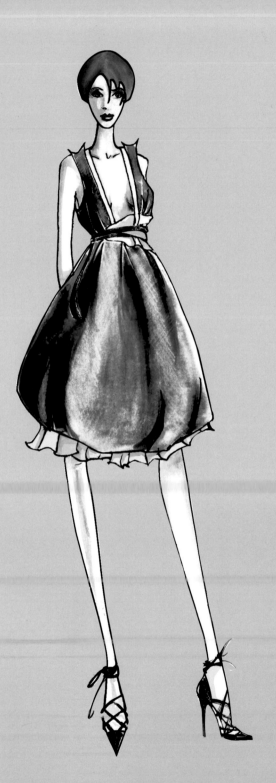

Romantic warrior theme

To accentuate a glimmering effect, use a fixative which allows the colours to fuse into one another. Once the fixative is dry, it is advisable to retrace the outline as it will have faded slightly.

FABRICS

PHRYNÉ
PUFF BALL COCKTAIL DRESS WITH PLUNGING SQUARE NECKLINE. PLEATED GODET SKIRT UNDERNEATH ECHOING THE INLAID FABRIC OF THE HIGH-WAIST AND BELT. HIDDEN BACK FASTENING.

Layering and colour rendering using Photoshop

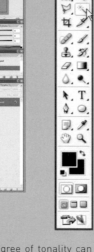

Once the silhouette and the fabrics have been scanned, open them up in Photoshop.

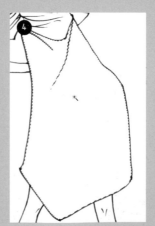

The speed in which this computer work can be executed largely depends on the quality of the original drawing. It is important to make sure that the outlines of the garments are a continual line without any gaps. It is not an absolute rule but, in this case, it will greatly facilitate the project. Once all the checks are done, scan the drawing to a suitably high resolution. Here the drawing has been scanned to 600 dpi. Scan the chosen fabrics onto the illustration with the same resolution. A high resolution scan can even show the weave of fine fabrics.

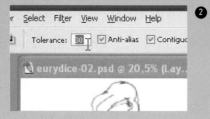

The degree of tonality can be determined by using the tolerance parameter. The greater the tolerance value the greater the selected area is. For example, an 0 value is equivalent to an area of a few pixels, whereas a 100 value represents a much larger area.

Now use the magic wand tool, found in the toolbox, to select the areas on the illustration where you wish to overlay the fabrics. This magic wand allows you to select areas of colour with the desired tones.

> A numeric image shows information concerning the resolution. This defines the degree of detail which will be represented on the image. (The resolution is determined at the moment it is numbered and when it is printed.) An image's resolution is defined by the number of pixels in relation to a unit of length. It is expressed in dpi (dots per inch in English) or ppp (*pixels par pouces*, in French).

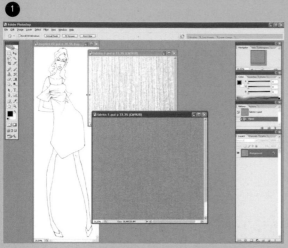

Set the tolerance parameter to 20, then select all the areas on the dress by clicking inside the outline. These areas will become highlighted as is shown in the diagram to the left. To add another area to the selection, use the upper case key on the keyboard. A little sign ←← - →→ will appear. Attention: if the selected area is clicked accidentally, it will become 'deselected'.
It is also possible, even recommended, to use the Zoom icon in the Toolbox to show up small areas which are not noticed on a larger scale: by doing this, nothing else will be altered. You can then zoom in and out, as desired, then use the magic wand to complete the selection.

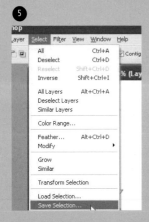

All that is necessary then, is to click and drag the fabric image over the illustration document.

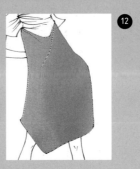

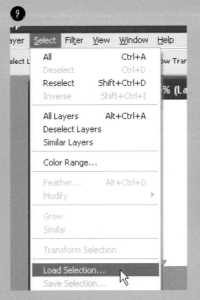

To be able to use it afterwards, save this selection by clicking on the Select menu and in the drop down menu, click Remember/Memorise

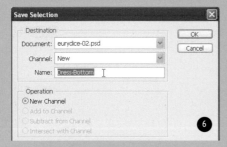

A dialogue window will then appear. In the Name field, type in the title of this selection, then click on the OK button to confirm. Repeat this process of selecting and saving for the other parts of the garment.

To aid the rest of the process, take care to select the bottom, middle and top of the skirt. You will then have, in this example: the « dress » selections, « bottom-dress », « middle-dress », « top-dress », and « bands ».

A new layer is created automatically. Reselect the previously saved dress selection and press the Invert mode. (figs. 9,10,11) This will have the effect of selecting everything that is outside of this area or zone, then press the Remove (or Delete, or Backspace) key to remove the fabric which is outside the dress outline (fig.12)

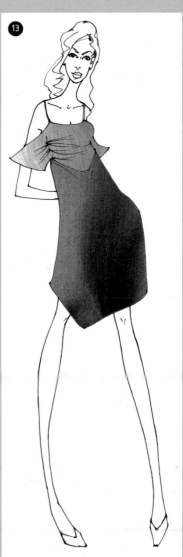

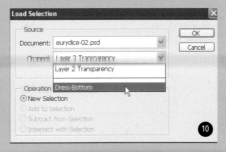

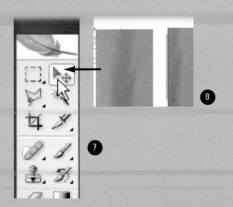

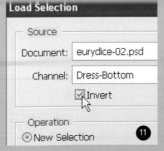

Once this has been achieved, the fabrics can be imported into your document. This is a simple operation: just select the document, containing the fabric, open at the same as the illustration (click on this image to open the document), then choose the Move icon in the toolbox.

Repeat the same operation to overlay the bands of fabric as seen in fig.13.

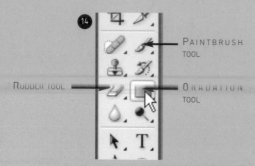

PAINTBRUSH TOOL

RUBBER TOOL

GRADATION TOOL

To develop the work further and give the illustration a bit of volume, make use of different tools such as the Gradient (for the colour), Paintbrush and Rubber icons.

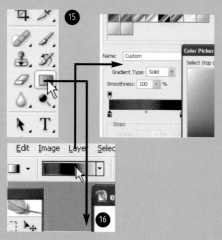

The first stage consists of giving a general volume to the dress. Use the Gradient icon found in the toolbox. By selecting this icon, a dialogue box appears under the menu bar (fig.15). Click on the button indicated by the mouse, the Gradient window opens (fig.16).

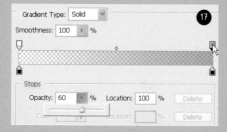

Using the different colour and transparency parameters/fields (fig.17) a personalised gradation can be created. The small cursers situated above the gradation bar control the transparency, the ones below, the colour. An indefinite number of cursers can be inserted whether it be for colour or transparency.

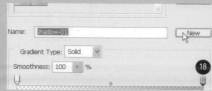

Finally, it is important to safeguard the newly-created gradation by naming it then click on the New button to validate it (fig.18).

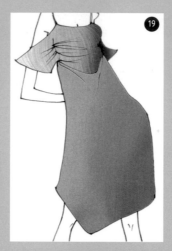

Once the gradation parameters/fields are saved, close the dialogue box to return to the illustration. Before applying the gradation, you will need create a new layer in which the previously saved 'dress' selection will be found (figs. 9 and 10). The gradation will only appear in the selected area. Click once with the tool to define the start of the gradation. By moving the mouse, the length and direction of the gradation can be decided. It is equally possible to start and finish on the inside as well as on the outside of the selected area in order to add shading. Having gradated the dress, the gradation of the dress bands can be added (fig.19) following the same process and creating another layer to add the shadows.

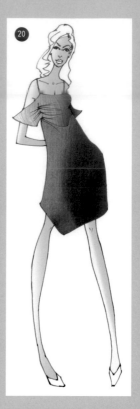

This same system can be applied to apply gradation to the skin and hair colours, and accessories in your illustration, providing the following steps are taken:
1- Select the area on the overlay of the illustration drawing.
2- Create a new layer and apply the gradation onto it.
3- Create a new layer for each new gradation, then, when satisfied with the result, fuse the different layers all together to obtain one single layer. In the example shown here, there are seven different layers merged into one!

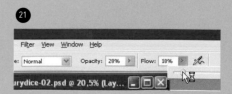

At the finishing stage, once everything is saved, the work can be refined by using the Paintbrush and Rubber tools to adjust the volume, if necessary. When using the Paintbrush, the ink flow parameters can be defined (similar to using an airbrush) – this means transparent colours strokes can be corrected using the Rubber.

COLOUR WAY

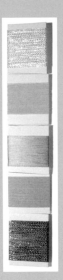

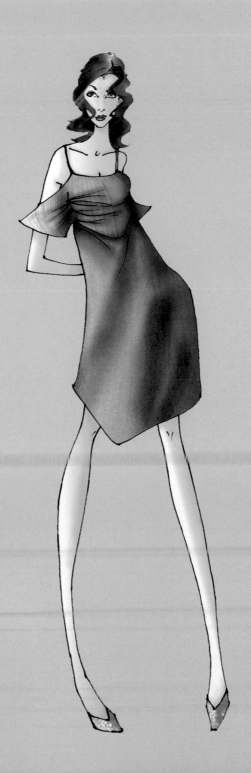

Ode to a rose
theme

FABRICS

EURYDICE
OFF-THE-SHOULDER SHORT-SLEEVED DRESS HELD UP BY STRAPS.
SLIGHTLY FLARED WITH HIGH-WAIST UNDER THE BUST. INVISIBLE
BACK FASTENING.

applying flat colour using Photoshop

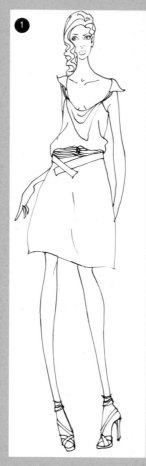

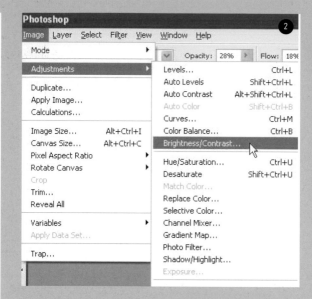

A quick, easy and most frequently-used way of giving life to a drawing is to apply colour using the flat method. In the absence of a realistic effect, this technique gives a very good idea of colour harmonies to the outfit.

> The contrast of a drawing depends on the number of tones used between the white and the black. The stronger the contrast, there are less grey tones. By increasing the contrast in your drawing, the rest of your work will be made easier.

Scan the illustration into Photoshop taking care to contrast the drawing using the Brightness/Contrast function in the Image menu.

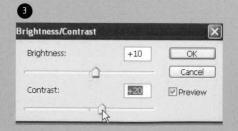

To add colour, the main part of the work is to separate out the different areas which make up the garment on the different overlays. If they do not appear on the screen, they can be found in the Window menu, or by pressing the F7 key on the keyboard.

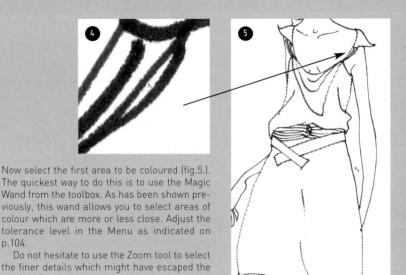

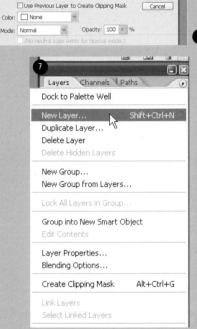

Now select the first area to be coloured (fig.5.). The quickest way to do this is to use the Magic Wand from the toolbox. As has been shown previously, this wand allows you to select areas of colour which are more or less close. Adjust the tolerance level in the Menu as indicated on p.104.

Do not hesitate to use the Zoom tool to select the finer details which might have escaped the eye (fig.4).

Once a selection has been made, you will make a new layer on which the colour can be applied. Go to the Layer menu and click on the little arrow in the top right of the layer window (fig.6.)

Name each of the layers as this will help you quickly identify which elements correspond to which (fig.7).

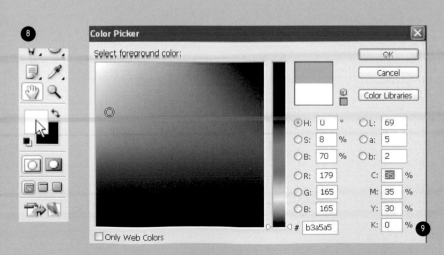

You can now proceed to the colour selector. By using the colour selector, erroneous interpretations can be avoided. However, there is also a difference between the colour on the screen and that which is printed. Various factors determine this, i.e. type of paper or ink used, printer quality etc. We suggest using the Pantone R references – these are universally-used colours, whichever the industry.

To choose a colour, click on the foreground colour in the Toolbox (fig.8). The dialogue window of the colour picker will then appear (fig.9).

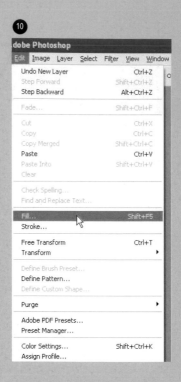

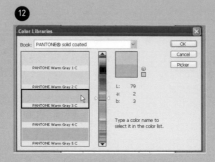

The last stage consists of filling the selected area with your chosen colour (on a new layer). To do this click on the Fill button in the Edit menu (fig.10).

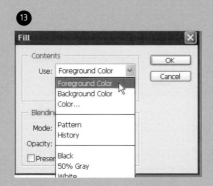

Once the dialogue window in Fill appears, take care to select the foreground colour!

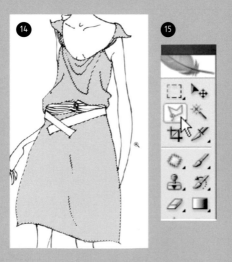

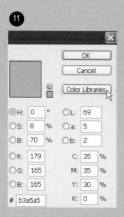

Finally the area is filled with your chosen colour (fig.14). All that is left to do is to repeat the process for the remaining areas.

Following the same principle, it is possible to apply volume to the garment by creating shadows. This is done using the polygonal Lasso tool (fig.15) and selecting the area to be filled with a darker or lighter colour.

Choose a colour from the palette, then click on the Colour Libraries button. The Pantone shade will appear with the colour, and reference, of your choice.

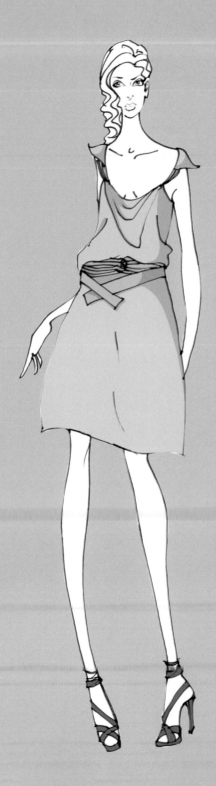

Ode to a rose
theme

FABRICS

HELENE
FANCY-STRAPPED DRESS, SLIGHTLY FLARED WITH A DRAPED NECK-
LINE AND INLAID BELT. HIDDEN BACK FASTENING.

The merchandiser compiles a collection plan which is more commercial than the one destined for the press and professionals.

The design team complete, or adapt, certain items and detail them in what is known as a style book.

In response to the demand of the textile industry or distributors, the targeted catalogues are further developed by an independent style bureau whose job, amongst others, it is to determine the trend with its corresponding products. One of their services is to offer sourcing with forecasting studies. The proposed items will be used as they are or reinterpreted by licensed partners.

In the case of licences, the catalogues are developed by designers in licensing offices. Although they have a tendency to disappear, largely due to a fear that the brands will ultimately have more control over the image, their job is to finalise the coordination of the different collections and lines using the brand.

In this chapter we detail the contents of these catalogues necessary for the manufacture, commercialisation and distribution of fashion items, paying particular attention to the quality of their organisation and presentation. We have taken the opportunity to explain how to compile a similar book. In fact, it is very important that a young designer is capable of producing the latter, in the same way as he, or she, does a curriculum vitae, as it will become a vital part of the project.

The books we present here have been inspired by those produced in studios which offer a series of coordinated products between them. It must contain all the information necessary to facilitate a good understanding of styling. This personalised and focused book must demonstrate, in general terms, your style to future working partners.

Thanks to computers, it is much easier today to compile a portfolio which enhances the value of a product line and its contents. The visual impact of a catalogue depends on two essential factors: primarily, a good scheduling of the outfits is required i.e. overview, or page layout, development and secondly, specific graphic aspects, such as the choice of dominant colour choices, logo treatment and page setting.

This chapter explains how to develop an efficient house style and define a brand-identity. The organisation of this visual presentation must in fact demonstrate a unity which fully responds to the concept.

This book lists all the costs incurred in a commercial collection by detailing all the products. It also contains technical and thematic information relative to these items, for example:

- seasonal indications for the year (spring-summer or autumn-winter);
- the themes, depicted on the mood boards, which reveal the various sources of inspiration;
- the details of the product collection, which have been developed to identify the brand and season;
- colour ranges and harmonies, shown by theme and through each product item;
- the silhouettes, which establish the balance between the products and their volume;

- the collection plan organised by categories (shirts, tops, dresses, jackets, trousers, etc.);
- the fashion illustrations, which propose the coordination of the products, accompanied by colour swatches and fabric samples;
- finally the shapes on the dress form, or tailor's dummy, enabling the modellers to interpret the designer's ideas as close as possible;
- precise indications regarding the manufacture of the items

As we have seen in the introduction, these books have several uses, not least, it serves as a very useful communication tool between the brand and the various manufacturers, as is illustrated below.

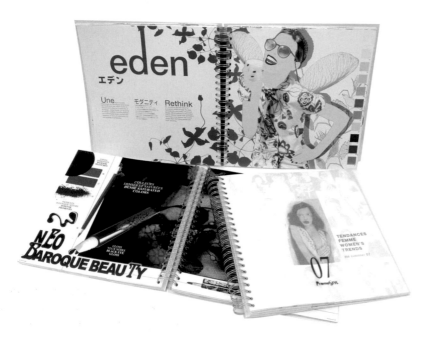

Cover and inside pages of a 'promostyle', spring-summer 2007 – a women's trend book. on the cover the title features as does the season and the target. the double theme page 'eden' includes a small piece of presentation text, a fashion illustration showing a printed blouse and its colour range. the cosmetic page describes a range of make-up suitable for the colour theme. You will notice that the colour range used for the cosmetics (powders, lipsticks, eye shadows) are done in the same manner as the fabric samples.

House brands

A *prêt-à-porter* brand uses different manufacturers, each with their own speciality, making only one type of product: knitwear, dressmaking, suits or leather. Here the information, established by the design team, will assist in understanding the collection in its entirety enabling a coherence of the different lines and the distribution sites.

These books are particularly important when the brand uses delocalised manufacturers, particularly those in the emerging countries such as India and China. The company, in this instance, economises on space and salaries, as there is no production studio to take into account. The prototypes are made by factory pattern cutters, then approved by a design team from the brand before being put into production. In this first instance, the designer's professionalism is essential to the success of the brand.

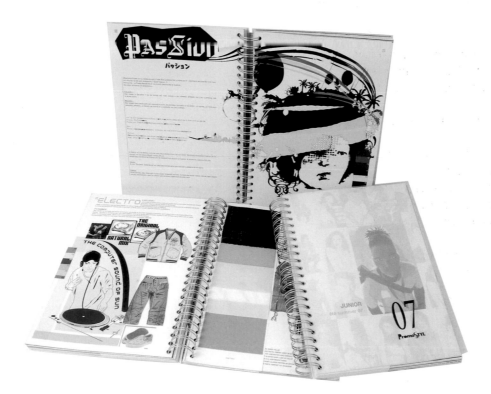

Cover and interior pages of the Junior Promstyl, Spring/Summer 2007 notebook. Above: a double-page spread with the theme 'Passion'. Left: a double-page spread presenting the basic products and sample colours.

The licences

In the licensing field, a team within an international licensing office of the brand and its designers, establish the books by product-type (men's, women's or children's *prêt-à-porter*, accessories; home and interiors). The collections are either used as they are or adapted to different markets by in-house designers under-licence, making sure the brand-identity is respected: before distribution, all the modified products must be approved by the international licence office. Here again, the book serves as an indispensable support, guaranteeing that the brand's image is respected.

It should be noted that, in this case, the designer will more than likely have to visit the factories to make sure that the products are being made to the specifications detailed in the book.

The labels

In the textile industry, French or otherwise, a distributor such as Monoprix can call on design consultants such as Perclers Paris, Promostyl, or Nelly Rody to produce one or several collections presented under different labels.

This out-sourcing allows the company to significantly reduce salary costs as the in-house designers are not used.

Using the products books, supplied by the design consultants, the manufacturer will be able to make the prototypes, either for itself or for a distributor.

The portfolio

'Jazz' portfolio of Hanako Chiba, student
The trend defined here is associated with music and life style. The vinyl disc and the plastic cover evokes a past era, reinterpreted in a contemporary way, giving a new facet to nostalgia.

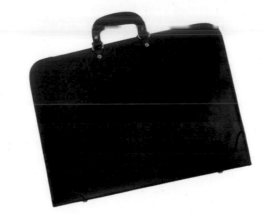

Portfolio

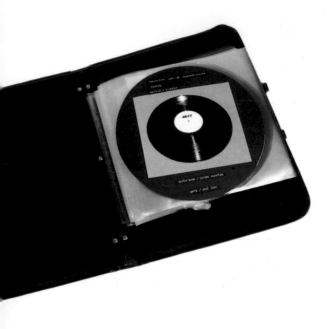

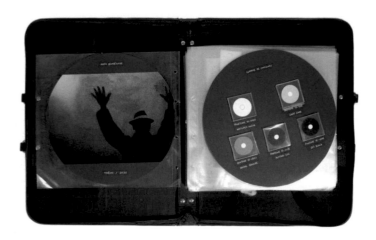

Title page. The choice of using a vinyl disc, rather than the New Orleans group itself for example, shows that it is more about evoking a mood linked to jazz than the culture from where it originates.

Mood page making reference to *Shadows*, a film by John Cassavetes of jazz in the 1950s. The presentation of the colour range is symbolic of the jukeboxes of that era.

A portfolio consists of personal projects as opposed to the product book aimed at industry. It is normally packaged in such a way as to give it a distinguished identity. As an example, we have chosen a portfolio which evokes a mood, or feeling, resulting in a trend-setting collection – in this case it is both musical and intellectual. This portfolio demonstrates the capacity to carry out iconographic research, the ability to analyse, as well as summarise it, by means of illustrations – all of which are essential qualities required by design consultants. In fact, consultants need designers who are capable of gathering a large number of elements around a theme (with the development of colour schemes and fabric swatches) in order to define the trends.

The portfolio must target the fashion sector which the designer has identified: luxury end, design, textile industry, design consultancy, fabric construction etc.

Following the chosen speciality, the accent will be put on the

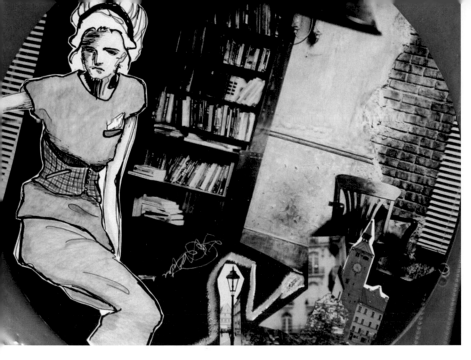

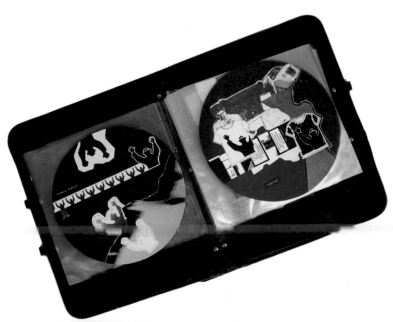

MOTIF VARIATIONS SHOWING A CONSISTENT DEVELOPMENT OF THE
MOOD OR FEELING.

illustration, fabrics, colours or the concept of the garment.
The elements which feature in the portfolio will be selected, in
relation to the target, from amongst the following:

- the text presenting the project/s;
- pages of captioned research images (to aid the understanding of the subject);
- fashion illustrations;

- product placing (suggesting moods, shop presentations);
- pages of fabric research and swatches;
- pages of colour schemes;
- pages of textile motifs and patterns;
- flat drawings with details and captions to help understand
  the garment.

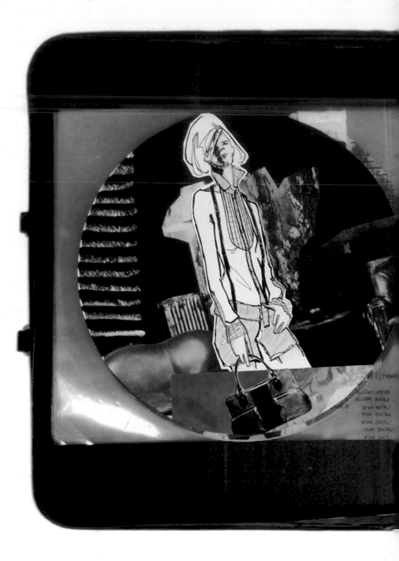

ILLUSTRATION SHOWING OVERALL 'LOOK'.

FABRIC PAGE SHOWING COORDINATED PRINTS FOR THE COLLECTION AND SOME DETAILS AND FINISHES. THE ILLUSTRATION CONFIRMS THE STYLE AND MOOD BY BALANCING THE PAGE.

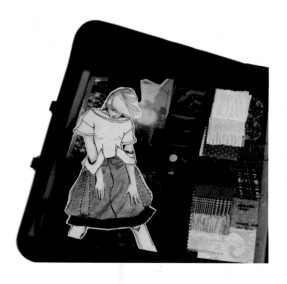

Good presentation of the portfolio is of the utmost importance, with particular care being paid to the graphics and coloured 'flats'. It is equally important to demonstrate a broad range of techniques which show the designer's strengths and knowledge. If the portfolio has been largely produced on a computer, it is an idea to do certain elements freehand as this will bring a richness and texture to the presentation, showing a sensibility for the materials.

Also, a coherent planning of the different elements will underline the designer's style (see the overview or layout diagram on the following pages).

The portfolio is the designer's world. Other than showing

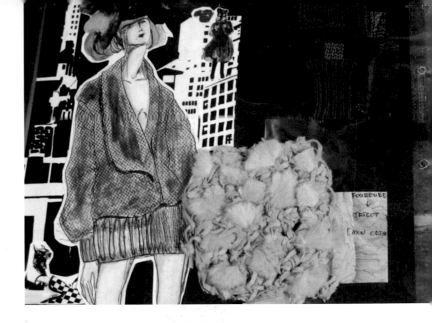

ILLUSTRATION SHOWING OVER-SIZED KNITTED CARDIGAN, WITH SAMPLES OF DIFFERENT STITCHES AND THREADS.

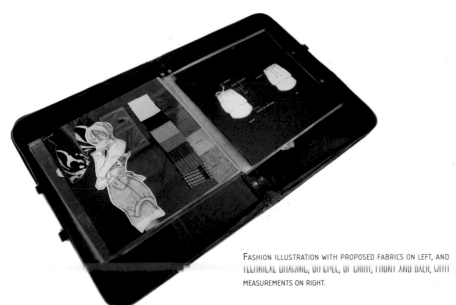

FASHION ILLUSTRATION WITH PROPOSED FABRICS ON LEFT, AND TECHNICAL DRAWING, ON LINE, OF GRAT, FRONT AND BACK, WITH MEASUREMENTS ON RIGHT.

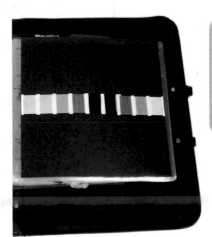

COLOUR SCHEME MADE FROM SILK THREADS. THIS COMPLETES THE RICHNESS AND TEXTURE OF THE 'GREE' DRAWINGS SHOWN PREVIOUSLY.

his or her savoir faire, it must reflect the culture of this milieu, i.e. make-up, hairstyles, fashion photography, styling etc. as well as aesthetic references, musicals, films etc. and his or her interpretation thereof. In fact, it is the designer's personal identity and his or her capacity to project this into the fashion world, which must come through in this book.

Before beginning a project, it is important to draw up a plan, which in this case corresponds to a layout sequence. This will include all the elements in your specifications book.

By establishing this system, your style book, portfolio or any aspect of your project is given a certain structure. It is the first stage of their construction. As with a book or a magazine, the work is presented in a logical manner which draws the reader's attention and gives the impression of a constant progression.

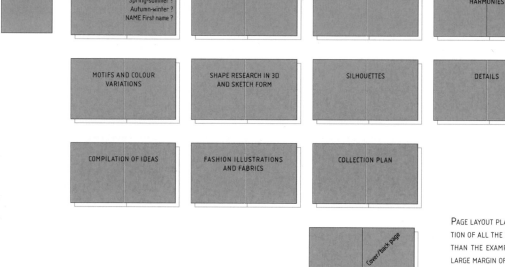

PAGE LAYOUT PLAN. VERY SUMMARISED, IT SHOWS THE ORGANISATION OF ALL THE ELEMENTS. HOWEVER, IT IS MUCH LESS DETAILED THAN THE EXAMPLE SHOWN ON THE OPPOSITE PAGE, LEAVING A LARGE MARGIN OF INTERPRETATION.

What is a layout sequence?

In the press and publishing world, a page layout is a schematic representation of all the pages making up a magazine, a newspaper or an illustrated book. In this case, it allows the illustrations to be distributed harmoniously throughout and gives the book a rhythm, as well as working out the number of necessary pages and work plan.

The page layout is arranged on one single sheet, so that the entire project can be seen immediately. Ideally, it should be hung on the wall so that it can be consulted at any time allowing for any inevitable modifications to be made as one goes along.

Structuring advice

The organisation of a portfolio must, above all, reflect a coherence of ideas from the designer. Do not present all your work under the pretext of showing everything you can do : too many exercises will look too much like a school-book. The portfolio is designed for professionals who will be judging your professionalism so strategies and assurances are necessary. It is preferable to choose a precise theme and rework certain elements that have been particularly successful. This can be done by selecting graphics which complement the idea, rather than juxtaposing a series of unrelated and disparate pieces of work. By the same token, an interesting element lost in a discordant presentation is likely to be considered accidental, rather than deliberate.

Therefore, begin by making a rigorous selection of the factors which best illustrate your design. Knowing how to compile a style book, successfully produce fashion plates, execute precise technical drawings are the vital elements which must be mastered. In the portfolio however, it is the relevance of your topic and style which will be the proof as to whether it is worth pursuing. The readers would like to be surprised by your acumen and professionalism.

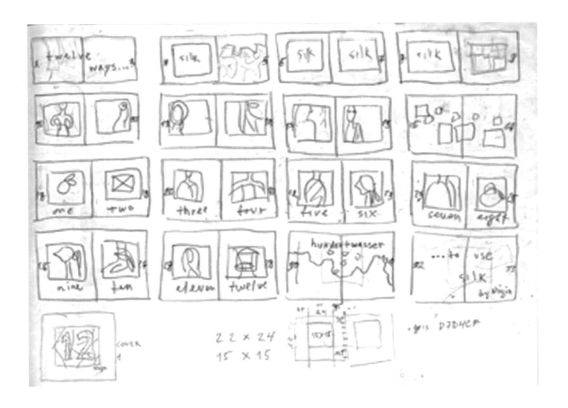

PAGE LAYOUT IN FORM OF A STORY-BOARD WITH ROUGHS GIVING
AN IDEA OF PLAN ALTERNATION (CLOSE UP, ZOOM, PLAN VIEW ETC.).
IT PROPOSES A CONCRETE IMAGE AND GIVES VITALITY TO THE PROJ-
ECT.

To summarise, the portfolio is the filter which demonstrates your ingenuity and captures the imagination of its reader because you stand out!

As a working tool, the product book deals with the practical demands of the project and will be organised in a more rigorous manner.

It is advisable to divide it into several parts or chapters. The first part introduces the subject: here you present the theme and the concept upon which you have based your ideas, as well as the shapes, colours and fabrics, mood pages, silhouettes, and finally details and finishes.

The second part consists of the design development with fashion illustrations, the products accompanied by technical information (larger plans of details, fabrics and model descriptions). We suggest that you present a fashion illustration on one page and, on the opposite, a technical drawing of the product, detail sketches (collars, sleeves, fastenings etc.), fabric samples, colour variations etc. The more detailed the technical information, the less difference there will be between the finished product and your original idea.

Finally, it is helpful to include an appendix to your work as this will assist in understanding the project. For example, this could include the origins of your idea, research on already existing products, and idea compilations up to your theme research. These supporting documents will give depth to your portfolio.

A final word of advice: it is better to have a project with a lot of pages and a small amount of information on each page than the contrary - this makes for much easier reading and comprehension.

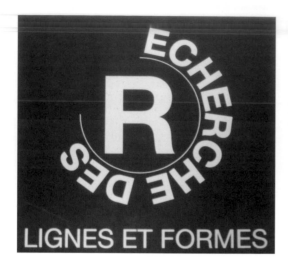

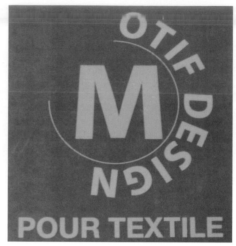

THE NAME OF A PROJECT CAN BE TREATED AS A LOGO. THESE TWO EXAMPLES SHOW GRAPHIC RESEARCH IN THE TRADITION OF THE VOLUME AND SHAPE STUDIES OF THE BAUHAUS, WHICH ILLUSTRATE PERFECTLY LINE AND SHAPE WORK.

TO PRESENT ANOTHER EXAMPLE USING A MOTIF, BUT KEEPING THE SAME HOUSE STYLE, THE BACKGROUND TEXTURE CAN BE ACCENTUATED BY LESSENING THE CONTRAST BETWEEN THE BACK AND THE FOREGROUND.

What is a house style?

After having organised the contents of your portfolio, you will then have to construct its visual impact by creating its house style. This is a document which appoints a set of visual norms or standards, to be used by a company, organisation or for a project. It defines the visual identity of the above and guarantees a coherent communication. House styles are devised for magazines, newspapers and television channels, advertising campaigns (television, cinema, the press, advertising hoardings etc.) and on the Internet ... so, in fact, every type of media. In the case of a product or brand, the house style insures a visual link between these different forms of communication.

A style book is also a visual communication document. By creating a house style before beginning the page layout work, it will immediately give you a backbone and unite your presentation, which in turn will help your efficiency.

The house style revolves around three complementary elements: the logotype (logo), the typography and the colours. All of these contribute largely to the overall feel of your chosen mood provided, of course, they are in keeping with your proposed theme, i.e. design, vintage, romantic, punk, etc.

Logos and brands

These are names, symbols, or other small designs, adopted by organisations to identify its products etc. as the following examples show: a logo can identify a company (Air France, Microsoft), a brand (Hermès, Louis Vuitton, Chanel) and even a product or product line of a brand (Nike Air, L'Oreal's Studio Line), as well as an institution (UNESCO, United Nations), a sporting manifestation (Olympic Games, Football World Cup) or a cultural event (Cannes Film Festival or the Golden Globe Awards). It is normally a name using a specific typeface placed in a particular manner. But this can be extended to a logo being just an image (sometimes a simple sign), the first letter of a name or an acronym. Brands such as Lacoste (with the crocodile) or Gucci (with the horse's bit) having been using their logos on

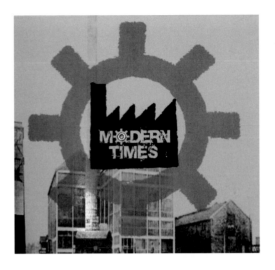

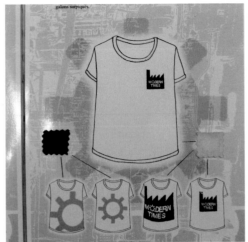

galons surpiqués

THE INDENTED WHEEL, EVOKING MACHINERY, THE DRAWING SYMBOLISING A
FACTORY, THE WEATHERED OUTLINES OF THE TYPOGRAPHY AND THE GENERAL-
LY BRUTALIST TREATMENT DEPICT THE THEME OF THIS BOOK: THE INDUSTRIAL
WORLD OF PREWAR AMERICA ILLUSTRATED BY THE CHARLIE CHAPLIN FILM

MODERN TIMES. YOU CAN COMBINE, AS SHOWN HERE, THE LOGO TEXT AND
BRAND NAME OR CLOTHING LINE. THE BRAND WILL BE ABLE TO BE USED IN A
VARIETY OF WAYS, LIKE HERE, WITH A PLACED MOTIF ON A TEE-SHIRT.

Creating a logo

their clothes and accessories for more than 50 years.

During the last two decades, it has become a basic identifying element with a lot of casual and sportswear brands, such as Nike (the tick), Adidas (three bands) and Quicksilver (the wave) whose designs have been based around it and, in some cases, the logo becomes more important than the clothing itself! The logo is also a distinctive sign of belonging to a particular group.

As a reaction, certain brands have adopted, for several years now, a type of reverse politics by not using any logo at all, e.g. American Apparel, Muji, or Nobrand. But, to communicate in this way, these brands still have to develop a house style which leads us to note that, amongst the three important elements, the logo is not the most important.

A logo is designed, most commonly, by a graphic designer. However, when used in conjunction with a clothing line, it is done in collaboration with the fashion designer. A good example of this is the collaboration between Yohji Yamamoto and the Adidas brand for the clothing line Y-3.

To personalise your project, you could design your own logo. Don't forget that there is a plethora of signage in everyday life such as signposts for airports, for example, which are simple yet immediately understood. These could serve as good starting points. Analyse the commercial message conveyed by logos in magazines or on advertising hoardings: your logo must demonstrate an organised thought process. The more explicit it is, the more it will be justified.

It is necessary to imagine this logo

in relation to the project theme and destination: clothing line, mood or personal presentation work. Numerous factors need to be taken into account such as the size of the letters, as well as the colours and shapes. As a general rule, a round-shaped logo will give the impression of security and well-being, triangular shapes will symbolise innovation and state-of-the-art technology and square shapes will evoke stability and sturdiness.

A logo can be a combination of an image and a word. Do not hesitate to have several attempts by arranging the text and image differently and altering their size until you arrive at a balanced composition.

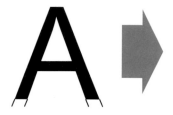

Arial, Helvetica, Univers, America Sans, ITC Avant garde, BiTDUST TWO, Blue Highway, bubble boy, Myriad, Isonorm, df667 chlorine, Blippia, BLOCKOUT, Alba, ...

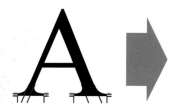

Times New Roman, **Albertus MT**, ARSIS, Bitstream Vera Serif, Book Antiqua, Cantabile, City D, Courrier, Garamond, IM FELL DW Pica, Palatino Lynotype, **STENCIL STD**, ...

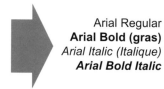

Arial Regular   Corps 08
Arial Bold (gras)   Corps 10
Arial Italic (Italique) Corps 12
Arial Bold Italic   Corps 24

The letters

Typography is an essential element of any house style. It originated with the printing industry in the 15th century as the art of assembling letters to form words, phrases and texts. Typographic letters are classified into typefaces (Arial, Helvetica, Garamond etc.), which correspond to style of alphabet and are composed of different fonts (bold, italic, different sizes etc.).

The typefaces themselves are regrouped into families of letters (11 in total, according to the international classification Vox-Atypl used by professional graphic artists.

Here we present a simplified classification in two families, Serif font, meaning there are non-structural details on the ends of some of the strokes, and Sans Serif font, meaning those without. This is done to guide you through the innumerable typefaces which exist.

There are a lot of Internet sites entirely dedicated to typography and it is possible to freely download a number of typefaces (www.dafont.com for example). All you have to do is ensure that the typeface you choose is compatible with your software. (However, the majority of typefaces used nowadays are compatible with Mac's as well as PC's) and to copy the files «nomdelapolice.ttf» in the listings «/Library/Fonts» for Mac OS X or «C;\WINDOWS\ Fonts» for Windows.Windows.

HERMÈS

Dior   YVES SAINT LAURENT

DOLCE & GABBANA

Calvin Klein

CHANEL

THE TYPOGRAPHY OF THESE FAMILIAR BRANDS CULTIVATES A CERTAIN IMAGE OF ELEGANCE. THEY USE SIMPLE, SOBER AND TIMELESS TYPEFACES, IN PARTICULAR FOR AN ELEGANT THEME. AVOID FANCY TYPEFACES WHICH WILL COMPLETELY CONTRADICT YOUR PROJECT. A VERY DISTINCTIVE TYPEFACE CAN APPEAR OUTDATED VERY RAPIDLY.

Choice of typeface

It is strongly advisable not to use too many different typefaces as you will lose readability: three maximum will suffice. The first one is used for the titles. Select one that corresponds to your theme. For example, for a classic, elegant theme choose a simple, sober type face such as Arial, Tahoma or Helvetica; for a punk theme, a deconstructed design could work, or one which looks like it has been eroded by chemicals such as Got Heroin, Broken 15, Depraved; for a psychedelic theme, typefaces used on record sleeves of that era could work, such as Fillmore, Bell Bottom Laser, Butterfield.

It is possible to choose another typeface for the sub-titles. However, you could just alter the size of the one which you have just used for the titles. Finally, for the text, legends and captions, use simple ones such as Arial, Helvetica, Times, Myriad, Tahoma etc. If the more unusual typefaces work well for your titles and sub-titles, stick to the simpler-styled ones for long texts as these have to be read and not deciphered!

As a general rule, avoid eccentric and fancy typefaces. In preference, use simpler ones which, most importantly, work in conjunction with your theme. As is often the case, sobriety and simplicity is synonymous with elegance.

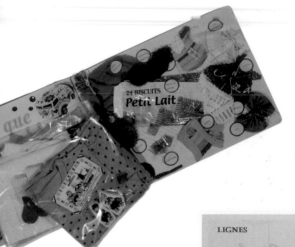

USE BRIGHT, GAY COLOURS FOR A CHILDREN'S CLOTHING PROJECT. NOTE THAT THE COLOUR SAMPLES AND FINISHING DETAILS ADDED PROVIDE COLOURED AREAS WITHIN THE BOOK. THEIR POSITIONING WILL HELP TO BALANCE THE PAGES.

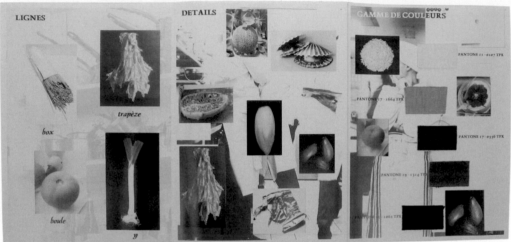

ON THIS SPREAD, THE EMPTY SPACES PLAY A VERY IMPORTANT ROLE AS THEY HIGHLIGHT THE COLOURS WHICH HAVE BEEN CHOSEN TO ILLUSTRATE THE 'FOOD' THEME. THE IMPACT OF THE NATURALLY BRIGHT COLOURS REINFORCE THE NEUTRALITY OF THE BACK-GROUND.

Colour is the house style factor which will have the most impact on the mood of your presentation. From the physical point of view, colours have differing wavelengths of light which are measured in microns. The human eye can only distinguish the light waves ranging between 400 and 700 microns. The colours which have the longer wavelengths are the biggest, therefore they are perceived more quickly. For example, reds (600-650 microns) give the impression that they are jumping out at you, whereas blues, with less microns (460–480 microns) are more soothing.

Symbolically, colours are associated with different concepts and meanings depending on the era and the place. For example, white, which in the West is associated with purity, innocent and peace is, in fact, the colour of mourning in Asia.

So that there is harmony between your choice of colours and project, we recommend that you use the ones from your colour range or palette. Generally, however, a neutral background is often the best means of emphasising your work.

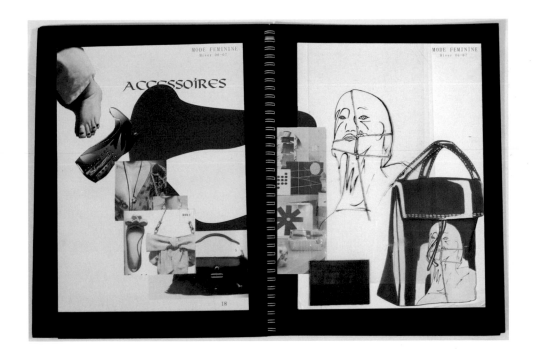

Neutral tones, like the white here, accentuate the vivid coloured areas giving a vitality to the reader. The black background paper plays an equally interesting role: by giving a contrasting effect, one is obliged to look at the centre of the composition.

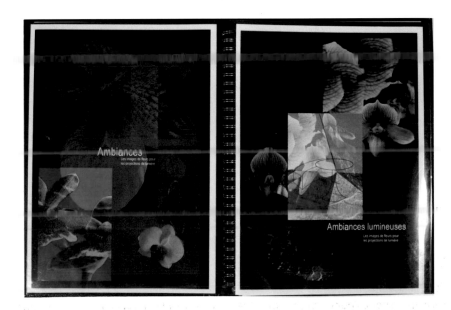

Black, particularly in the fashion world, conveys an image of elegance, luxury, modernity, as well as, mystery. This is particularly well-portrayed in this double-page spread.

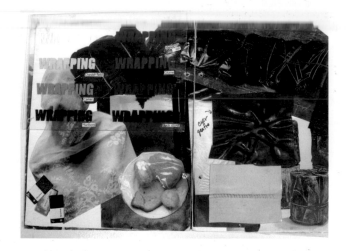

MOOD EVOKED. THIS HARMONIOUS COMPOSITION OF PLANES OF INSPIRATION, SHOWING A COLLECTION OF MATERIALS, INCLUDES UP TO FOUR DIFFERENT PLANES. USING A SHEET OF PERSPEX, ON WHICH THE TEXT HAS BEEN STUCK, ACCENTUATES THE RELIEF. THE ORGANISATION OF THE DIFFERENT PLANES GIVING A WEALTH OF INFORMATION TO THE PAGE.

The page layout determines the overall impression of the project. If you have chosen to keep it generally subjective, it is very important to adhere to certain rules which will emphasise the work.

A successful page layout presents the contents of the document in a harmonious and logical manner. Reading it will be made easier if the blocks of text/ images and colours are balanced and contrasted.

The first rule to follow can be summed up in two words: clarity and style. And just as the words evoke, this also applies to page layouts.

The second rule, which is just as important, is that of coherence: your page layouts must echo the theme and mood of your project. You will need to choose a format, paper and type of illustration which corresponds to your theme. For example, for a rural theme, you could use textured paper and natural colours; for a jazz theme (such as in the example on p.116), you could opt for a round format and plastic-coated black paper reminiscent of the old vinyl records which could be bought at Saint-Germain-des-Prés. Whatever it is, you must avoid, at all costs, superfluous decorations such as little bits of ribbon which have been used simply 'to make it look pretty'. The elements which are presented must contribute to the understanding of the project and not detract.

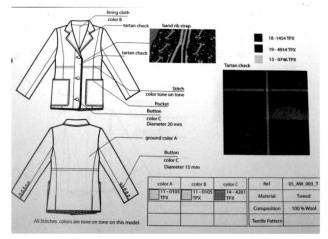

THIS SPECIFICATION SHEET SHOWS A 'FLAT' DRAWING OF THE FRONT AND BACK OF A JACKET, ACCOMPANIED BY THE NECESSARY EXPLANATIONS, CHOICE OF FABRICS AND PROPOSED PRINT. THIS HAS BEEN CARRIED OUT USING A COMPUTER AND, ALTHOUGH EXTREMELY PRECISE, REMAINS AESTHETICALLY PLEASING.

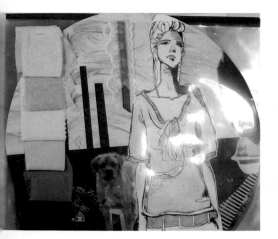

BY PLACING AN ILLUSTRATION UNDER A PLASTIC SHEET, IT SUGGESTS A PARTICULAR MOOD. THE MATERIALS ARE PRESENTED IN SUCH A WAY AS TO MAKE YOU WANT TO TOUCH THEM.

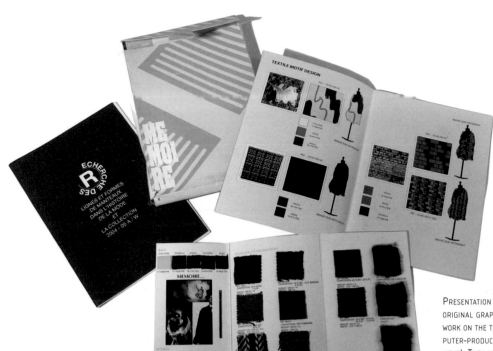

PRESENTATION PACKAGING (MADE AS A BOX, OR CARTON, WITH ORIGINAL GRAPHICS), TITLE PAGE (MENTIONED ON P.122) AND WORK ON THE TEXTILE DESIGN (WITH INSPIRATION PHOTOS, COMPUTER-PRODUCED MAQUETTES AND POSITIONING ON THE GARMENT). THE WHOLE PACKAGE IS VERY GRAPHIC, INCLUDING THE PAGE LAYOUT AND THE SUBJECT ITSELF. A WELL-STRUCTURED ORGANISATION HELPS THE READER. NOTE EQUALLY THAT THE FABRICS PRESENTED GIVE A RELIEF AND SUBSTANCE TO THE WORK.

Page composition

Following the layouts that you have already prepared (see p.120), you will have selected all the elements you wish to include page by page i.e. text, photos, illustrations, technical drawings, sketches and, of course, the fabrics. However, make sure that you do not consider the pages in isolation: they must interconnect with each other. Also, when one flicks through a book, it is not just one page, but two, that are seen at the same time. And so it is important to work on a double-page spread impact. Now, ask yourself the following questions: Which is the most important element to be presented on the spread? How do I emphasise it to catch the reader's eye? How do I attract his/her attention and make him/her follow my thought processes?

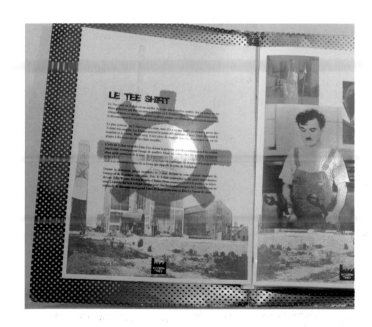

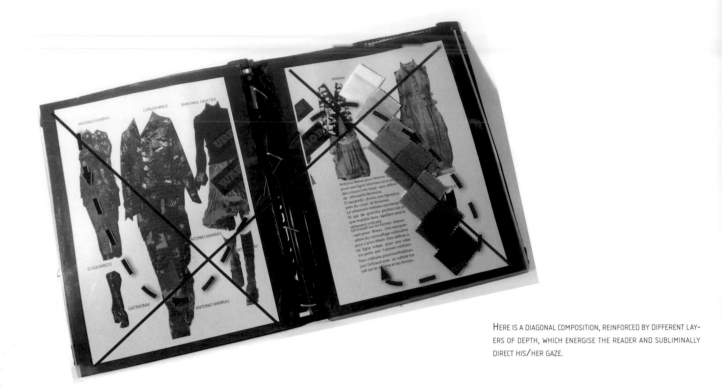

Here is a diagonal composition, reinforced by different layers of depth, which energise the reader and subliminally direct his/her gaze.

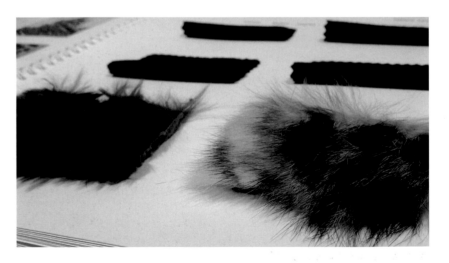

Additional fabric samples of your products are doubly interesting: they help the reader appreciate the textures whilst creating relief in your page layout, as is the case with these furs in the foreground.

Composition advice

- Each double-page spread of your project offers a visual unity, the composition of which can be likened to the work of a painter or photographer. It is necessary therefore to imagine the lines of composition around the blocks of text or image, and which ultimately guide the reader. Note that a diagonal composition will give the impression of movement and energy, whereas a horizontal, or vertical, composition will seem more measured and calmer.

- Make sure that the different blocks are equally spread out in order to balance the pages. Their positioning must guide the reader naturally. Look at

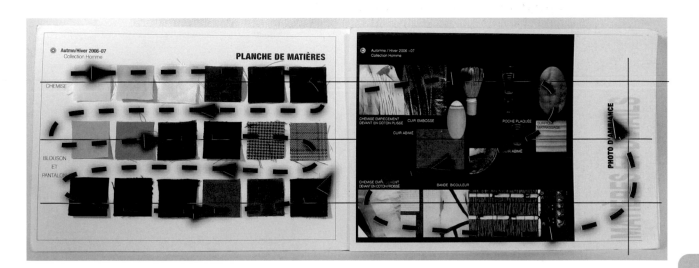

THIS SPREAD SHOWS THE SAME BALANCE BETWEEN THE ORGANISA-
TION OF THE FABRICS, ON THE LEFT, AND THE VISUAL INSPIRATION
PAGE, ON THE RIGHT. THE RESULT IS A FEELING OF GREAT SOBRIETY.
THE EYE FALLS NATURALLY ONTO THE RIGHT-HAND PAGE THEN FOL-
LOWS ONTO THE LEFT, READING FROM THE TOP TO THE BOTTOM AND
FROM RIGHT TO LEFT, LIKE WITH WESTERN WRITING.

fashion magazine advertising to inspire you. They are always composed in such a way that we notice the two most important things: the product and the brand.

- Think about altering the size of the letters and images in order to prioritise the information and emphasise the details which you judge to be important. It will be necessary to increase certain ones, decrease others, or superimpose them to create different planes.

At the same time, you will be able to create depth and rhythm to your spread.

Leaving the margins, or bleeding the page, gives the impression of depth and creates a certain movement.

- Placing elements across the two pages (a title, an image) links them visually.

- Do not overload the pages, too many elements will make the composition look confused.

- If you use a background image on one page, make sure it does not affect its readability.

- Finally, do not make your presentation too automatic/systematic. This can lull

the reader into a boring rhythm. On the contrary, create surprises which will constantly renew his/her interest. Whilst still adhering to the basic principles you have chosen for the presentation, consider changing the rhythm of your compositions, for example, from one chapter to another. Bearing in mind, however, that the technical part of your portfolio must be as clear as possible so as to be easily understood.

Portfolio of work

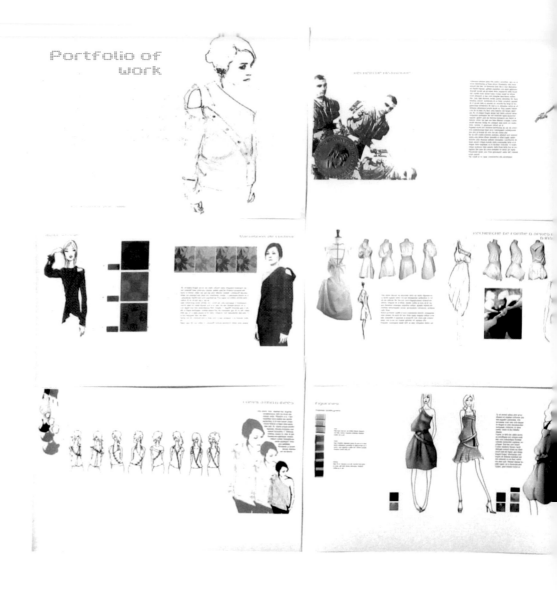

Looking at your work as you go along whilst the project progresses is essential as it will allow you to judge the balance within your portfolio. It is a question of placing your double-page spreads side by side, in the page order indicated by the layout. Attach them to the wall with masking tape, take several steps backwards then slightly narrow your eyes.

By doing this you will be able to notice any faults in the choice of colours, fabrics, typography, information prioritising and the absence or the redundancy of certain elements. It is important to look critically at your work; by doing this often, you will be able to train your eye. Do not hesitate to ask someone else's opinion, as they will be removed enough to evaluate the coherence of the project.

Amongst fashion magazine editors, this work irons out and

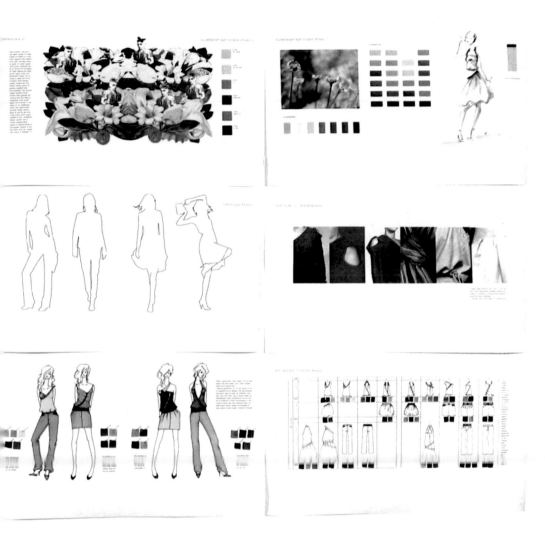

corrects the imbalances between the editorial departments (those who work on the magazine's house style) and the advertising departments, who must, despite their differing work remits, be able to integrate harmoniously to produce the magazine.

The fashion magazines are a good example to follow, for they are always produced in an interesting and attractive manner. A design student must practise this type of research regularly so that he/she can identify and understand perfectly certain constants evident in the presentation. In fact, the fashion world possesses its own codes of communication, visible in the treatment of current events whether it be artistic, architectural, musical, sport, economic or social – are usually the main topic headings in fashion magazines.

This chapter details the internal organisation of a design studio and its relationship with the other services of the *prêt-à-porter* business, giving the reader an insight into the work of a designer. A collection cannot be improvised. What is more, professional designers must not isolate themselves in their creative world and ignore the realities of the textile industry and the fashion market. The success of a great fashion designer is linked to their profound knowledge of the latter. Karl Lagerfield, for example, has demonstrated his creative genius to great benefit with brands such as Chanel, Lagerfield Galerie and Fendi and by respecting the individual image of each one, he has managed to compile truly original and distinctive collections.

If the production of the style book for the companies under licence, stays within the studio, they are principally centred on creating or designing. Essentially, they are dedicated to a choice of themes, to the definition of concepts, and the development of the collections (see Chapter 3). It consists of teamwork, where designers and different consultants, under the eventual authority of a creative director, work together by combining their skills: the design studio is a lively, versatile place where ideas circulate freely. Designers, like artistic directors, generally work on a freelance basis. They are normally linked to a company by the terms of a joint contract for a variable length of time, which can be extended for several seasons.

Over the past ten years now, new technologies have modified the organisation of the work within the studio. This has meant there is a quicker communication between the different services in the company, as well as with the suppliers and exterior consultants, who no longer have to move around as frequently.

The professional designer works in close collaboration with the *toiliste* who makes the collection's prototypes. This is why a good understanding of all the manufacturing constraints is necessary, so that he/she can be fully informed about the possible choices concerning finishes and fabrics.

In this chapter, we invite you to follow all the phases of development necessary for a collection by visiting the design studio and workroom, or atelier of the brand Lutz, which was created in 2000 by the designer, Lutz Huelle and his partner and financial director, David Ballu. To facilitate the understanding of the work of a workroom we have carefully broken down the

various modelling stages: first of all the draping, which consists of making the *toile* shape; developing the first *toile*, truing and checking the balance, trying the model on, pattern making, (that is to say the transfer of the different pieces from the *toile* onto a pattern card); and finally the cutting and assembling of these pieces into a garment.

At the end of this chapter, you will find the explanations necessary for the technical, or specification, drawings which make up the basis of the modeller's work. This type of 'flat' representation requires a complete understanding of the garment. The precision of the model's proportions, and suggested volumes, is paramount to guarantee a clear interpretation by the atelier. The flat drawings are also an essential element for the eventual production of a series.

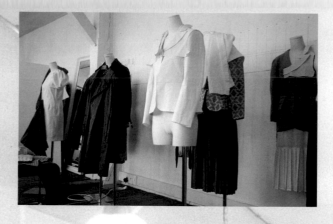

The team

The number of people working in a studio will vary depending on the structure and financial situation of the company. The team can be supervised by a creative director, as in the case of Alber Elbaz with Lanvin, Marc Jacobs with Louis Vuitton, Jean-Paul Gaultier with Hermès, to name but a few ... and by a studio director, such as Françoise Plaud with Lanvin, Anne-Marie Munoz with Yves Saint Laurent, Rosemary Rodriguez with Thierry Mugler.... The team consists of one, or several, designers who specialise in certain areas such as patterns or accessories, or are responsible for the fabrics, assistants and student placements. And finally, a house model who, fulfilling the aesthetic demands of the designer by her modelling skills and movement, enables all the garments destined for the catwalk to be tried and tested.

This model, whose measurements do not correspond to those found on the high-street, serve as an inspirational role for the designer or artistic director. Her principal function is to verify the look, silhouette, fall of the prototypes and harmonise the proportions and volumes of the different items of the collection.

External consultants

The design studio will sometimes call on the help of a fashion editor for advice on a collection and an external contribution regarding fashion show styling (for a 'look' development see Chapter 6, p.173). Examples of this external advisory role have been played by Carine Roitfeld, chief editor of French *Vogue* since 2001, for Givenchy, with Babeth Djan of Numero, for Lanvin and Marie-Amélie Sauvet, designer and ex-editor of French *Vogue*, for Balenciaga.

A graphic designer will be used for the layout of the collection's promotional information such as invitation cards, catalogues and press packs.

Finally, depending on the collection's requirements, the studio will call upon a number of specialist workshops, or ateliers, such as pearl embroiderers with the Maison Lesage, Montex and Co. and Vermont and Co.; fine dressmakers with Maison Gripoix, Robert Goossens, Delphine Charlotte Parmentier; feather makers such as Lemarié; milliners such as Jacques Lecorre, Philip Treacy, Maison Michel; corset specialists like Mister Pearl, Maison Cadole; glass and crystal specialists such as Swarosky; furriers such as Yves Salomon, Saga, Furs of Scandanavia; knitwear manufacturers, metal suppliers, printed tee-shirt specialists etc.

The designer chooses the items from the manufacturer's archives or orders an original bespoke item directly linked to the collection's theme. The fabric and haberdashery suppliers can also produce original designs for the collection.

The fashion calendar

The studio's calendar is governed by the fashion shows. The two seasons, spring-summer (SS) and autumn-winter (AW) are presented, respectively, between July and October and January and March. The collections presented in July and January are often pre-collections; they herald the season and are destined for the large distribution groups, who place orders at this point. At certain periods, the designer can be working on the SS and AW collections simultaneously.

A work-planner assists in the organisation of the team's work. The first stage is the research phase. It begins in January for the SS, in July for AW, for the season of the following year, and generally stretches over a period of one to two months. The designer carries out research trends so that themes and colour palettes can be defined. Sources originate from current art and theatre events, daily news, Internet research, overseas travel, vintage inspiration, with visits to flea-markets, and shopping (see Chapter 1).

The second stage involves visiting trade fairs to select fabrics and haberdashery items for sampling.

The third stage, which normally corresponds to the third month, is that of the designing of the garments for the collection. These are represented by fashion plates with fabric swatches and /or flat drawings. The items can be either, organised in a collection plan, or presented as a fashion show image: in this case the different looks are sketched and then posted onto the wall.

At the fourth stage the prototypes

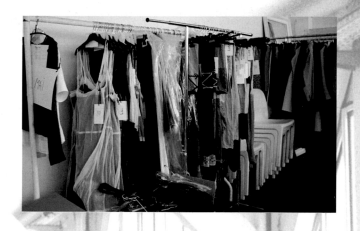

are launched. Here the design team works in close collaboration with the atelier technicians. The designer explains his/her drawings to the modeller and the prototypes are developed. When the atelier is overloaded with work, the designer will most probably outsource the work calling on a specialist studio to make the *toiles* and prototypes.

The fifth stage involves the designer preparing to present the collection to the company's commercial and press offices. Internal catalogues are developed where the drawings are cross-referenced with photos of the prototypes including the variations of fabrics and colours – all of which enable the commercial department to establish the costs. This 'bible' is shown simultaneously with the collection plan. Before the showroom sale, which coincides with the presentation of the pre-collection, the merchandiser chooses the looks and introduces them as photos and drawings into the commercial catalogue. This has the effect of drawing attention to certain products in particular.

Promotion and fashion show

Furthermore, the designer can organise shots for a photo-shoot (see Chapter 6, pp. 176-7). In this case, he/she will be taken to meet the photographers in order to establish a casting for the choice of models, as well as carry out an accessory styling. By collaborating with the photographer, the designer selects the shots and proposes a page layout maquette, which is eventually prepared by a graphic designer for the catalogue.

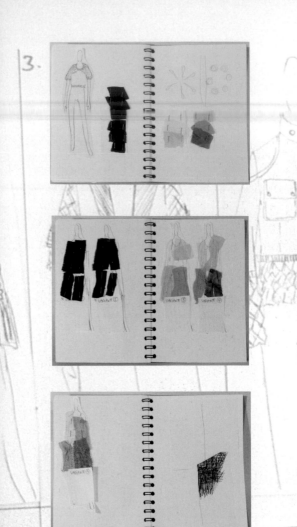

3.

5.

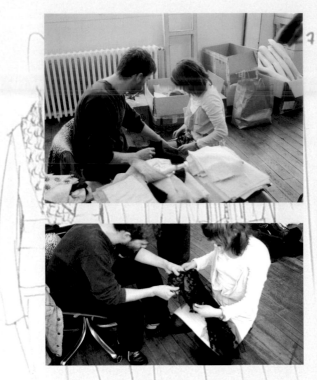

7.

Other work factors

Finally, unless he/she decides to use a production company who specialises in producing fashion shows, such as La Mode en Image or Alexandre de Betak etc., the designer proposes the feeling or atmosphere of the fashion show. This is done in collaboration with the production company, hairstylists and make-up artists. He/she can also choose the music and suggest the invitation cards. On the other hand, some designers prefer to use the services of a specialist design production company, such as Hervé Sauvage for example.

Design work also includes numerous brain-storming sessions and technical research trips. This research normally entails trips abroad to discover new manufacturers, specific product suppliers (baskets, hats etc.) and visits to trade fairs such as the Italian Le Linea Pele for leather, Moda in-Prato Expo for fabrics and Pitti Filati for knitwear.

Meetings with the brand's PR personnel are regularly scheduled to ensure that the collection's direction, commercial targets and brand image are all on course.

Finally, there are meetings with the financial department to establish the budget allocated to the collection – a consideration that the designer will have needed to have been aware of during the project.

The internal management of the design studio also plays an important role: the fabric and print samples need to be classified, the product drawings archived, as do the accumulated documentation such as magazines and books. During the course of the collections, this manner of archiving assists enormously

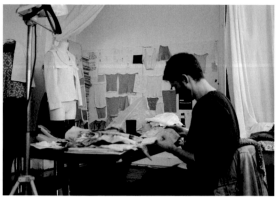

in creating a form of mini-library and information centre.

The studio assistants, amongst other things, tend to take care of the interior decoration of the studio by buying objects which relate to the collection's themes and contribute to the style and well-being of the studio.

The Lutz studio

For Lutz, shape research is a daily quest. Using his 'travel notebooks', he collects and catalogues information whilst in the street, on holiday, visiting exhibitions etc.

He also makes use of archives of his past collections, revisiting the details of previously-designed garments and breathing new life into them. Equally, his vintage clothing collection serves as a starting point, for he is able to adapt products and details and bring them up-to-date.

Finally, if all his collections have their own identity, Lutz writes what he calls a 'never-ending story'. Here, each

one becomes a supplementary chapter of history which expands, collection after collection. Witnessing the reoccurrence of certain ideas, notably the presence of knitwear in his collections, he admits he has an affinity with this. He prefers the freedom and infinite design possibilities it offers, as well as the technical savoir faire it requires, to the constraints of a finished woven material.

SHEET OF KNITWEAR FABRICS

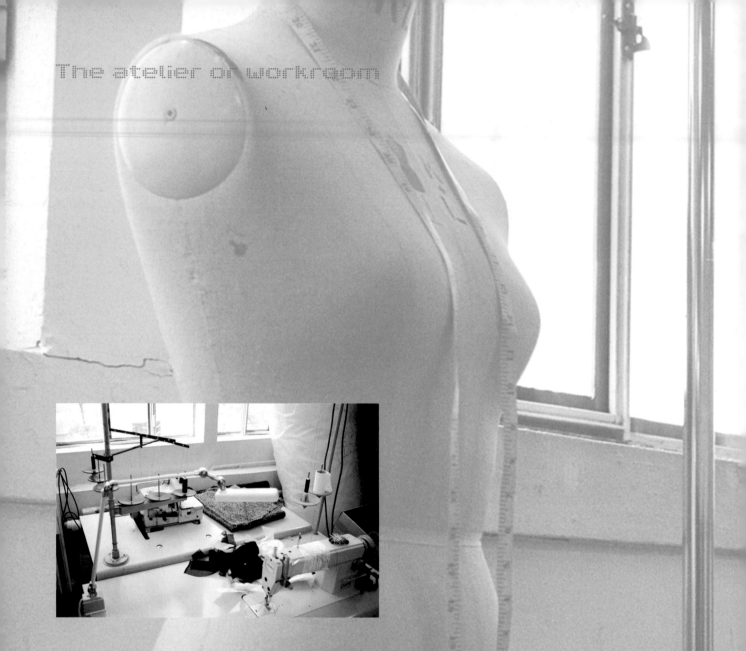

A number of different people work in the atelier. Namely the manager, one or two modellers who work from the designer's drawings, the sample machinists who make the prototypes and the students, who work there during the collection period. If it is an *haute couture* or luxury *prêt-à-porter* atelier, there is the addition of extra hands and specialist craftspeople.

The designer's success depends on the professionalism in his/her workroom. For example, it is in his/her best interest to allocate the work in relation to a particular field of expertise i.e. dressmaking, tailoring or knitwear so that they are dealing with familiar areas.

The atelier must be equipped with the appropriate materials in order to make the prototypes. In the absence of this, it will be necessary to call on the help of a design consultancy, or a specialised manufacturer equipped with the right materials and expertise to work in a particular area, for example with fur, leather, knitwear or lingerie.

Nevertheless, the designer must fully understand the workings of an atelier and be able to give clear instructions, so that the personnel are capable of interpreting the designer's wishes as closely as possible.

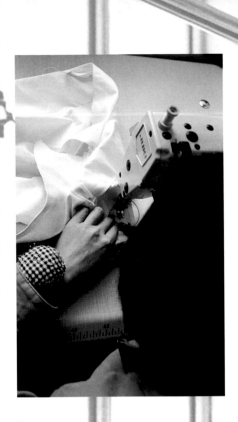

THE MACHINIST ASSEMBLES A PART OF THE *TOILE* ON HER SEWING MACHINE.

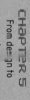

Daily communication between the designer and the atelier is of the utmost importance. During the collection period, the team will be required to make, what are sometimes, very difficult items. However good the drawings or well-researched the fabrics are, these will never substitute the reality. For there are occasions when fabrics react differently to what was expected and further research is required to finally develop the definitive model. The designer, therefore, might have to modify several pieces of the collection, and even abandon others, which the team have spent a lot of time working on.

An atelier must be clean, orderly and organised as the handling of particularly fragile fabrics demands discipline and care. The atelier is also a place of development for the *prêt-à-porter* items, standardising them according to the brand's different markets and communicating with the various production sites. It is also responsible for the initial model being adapted to the American and Asiatic markets, taking into consideration all the different morphologies that exist (see p.146). In this case, the costs linked to use of materials can be, in part, controlled. For example, the modeller will recommend the most economical way to position the pattern on the fabric. But, in other cases, such

désignation	fournisseur	rèférence	coloris	laize	qté/m/pc	qté total
tissus						
tissu	BELGOIE	LU3501 satin léger	99/noir	1,55	1,Σ	55
doublure	GOUMIEUX	LU300	99/noir	1,38	0,85	63,75
fournitures						
thermocollant	GLUTTY	NX1029	noir	1,5	0,2	15
gallon	GALONNADE	art.4430	noir		2,3	172,5
crochet	Captain	crochet	noir		1	75
zip/boucle	YKK	invisible	noir	35cm	1	75
façon						
façon modèle	CHIC COUTURE					
composition		51%SE 49%CO	100%AC		1	75
griffe					1	75
36						18
38						40
40						17
42						
44						75

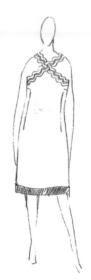

TECHNICAL PRODUCTION SHEET (ABOVE). IT LISTS THE FABRIC REFERENCES, STIFFENING AND LININGS, THEIR LENGTHS PER MODEL AND THE QUANTITIES TO BE ORDERED, BY COLOUR, FOR THE SEASON, AS WELL AS COSTING THE SUNDRIES. THE MODEL SKETCH, NAME AND REFERENCE AND SEASON INDICATION FIGURES AUTOMATICALLY.

R.HUM		LUTZ	
Saison 4-H 2006-2007		**Fiche technique de montage**	
	Croquis		**Description**

Couture: 1cn SAUF DEVOLTE /EMM = 0.5

Doublure: EN ENTIER → VOLANTE BAS FIXER TAILLE AVEC POINT LINGETTE

Surpiqure: NOIR ?
→ EMMANCHURE
→ DEVOLTE

NOTE BRETELLE → 1 = FIXER AU DOS ENTRE CORPS ET DECOUPETTE
2 = FINIR RABO

3 = APPLIQUER BRETELLES SUR DUT
→ LOTE DUT LES DOS DANS COUTURE LOTE + SURPIQUER
SURJET + APPLIQUER AU BAS DE LA COUTURE LOTE

BAS JUPE !! DOUBLURE
LOTON FOOT

Griffe: FLEUR DOS A 2.5 CM DU HAUT

Compo: COUTURE LOTE GAUCHE DOUBLURE
Taille: AVEC COMPO

(DF TH): BORD DEVOLTE SUR EMMANCHURE TAILLE +SUR CORPS

BIAIS TH:

TECHNICAL SHEET PRODUCED BY THE DESIGNER FOR THE *TOILISTE*. ALL THE FINISHES ARE DETAILED SO THAT THE PROTOTYPE CAN BE MADE AS CLOSE AS POSSIBLE TO THE INITIAL SKETCH.

as leather, it is the material which dictates the cut: a sheepskin only measures approx. 6 feet, i.e. six times 0.33 m² or 1.8 m²; the pieces are cut depending on its quality, i.e. quality A for the centre or 'flower', quality B for the chest area, and quality C for the sides (where numerous faults can be hidden).

When there are difficulties concerning a certain product, by way of a useful trick, Lutz uses pre-cut pieces, as well as sketches, to assist the *toiliste*. The toiliste makes a 'half-*toile*' in a fine plain weave made from a fine, medium or thick calico. The prototype is then made in a fabric, close to the final fabric, but not as costly (wool instead of cashmere, for example). Once the desired model has been achieved, it will finally be cut in the fabric chosen for the collection.

It is important to know that fashion show fabrics are 30% to 40% more expensive than the same fabrics used in production. This is because those, in the first case, are sold by the metre whilst those in the second (known as fabric pieces) are sold by the roll in 50 metres lengths.

To make a prototype, the fabric supplier delivers a length or 'sample length' which varies from 3 to 15 metres depending on the designer's needs, and of which the price is marked-up.

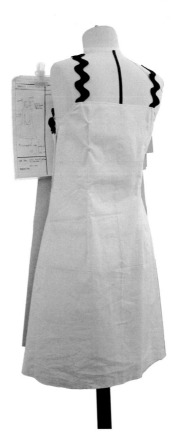

These pages show the first stage of model making where a *toile* is pinned onto the dress form. The toiliste prepares the pattern adding the seam allowances. From the *toile*, a rigid pattern card is made, then hung on the dress form. This is made up of the different pattern pieces, which will be cut out from the fabric and assembled to form the garment.

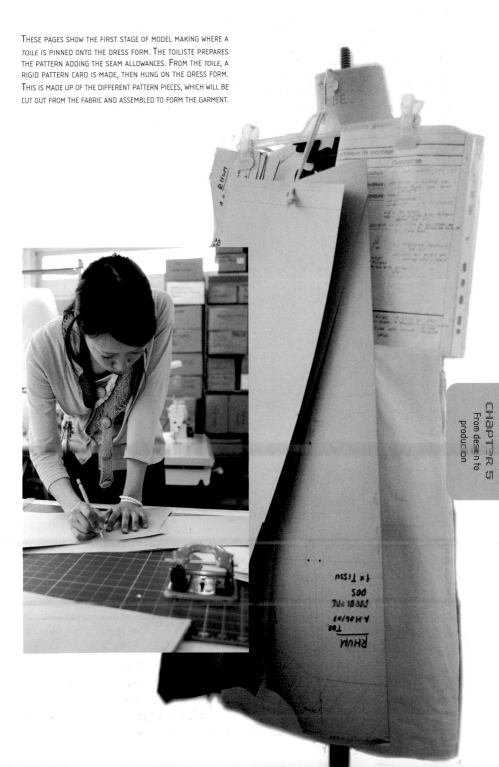

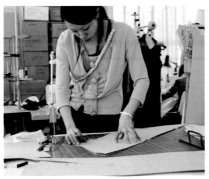

It is essential for the fashion designer to have a knowledge of body proportions. In spite of the differences in morphology, there are certain constants in measurements which determine the origin of standardised sizing.

MEASUREMENT CHART

MEASUREMENTS	SIZES				
	36	38	40	42	44
Nape to waist back	41,5	42	42,5	43	43,5
Neck to waist front	37	38	38,5	39	39,5
Waist to floor	105	105	106	107	108
Bust height	22,5–25,5	23–26	23,5–26,5	24–27	24,5–27,5
Half cross bust	9	9	9,25	9,5	9,75
Half bust girth	42	44	45	47	49
Half waist girth	31	33	35	37	39
Half hip girth	44,5	46,5	47,5	49	50,5
Half neck girth	17	17,5	18	18,5	19
Half back width across back	17,5	17,75	18	18,25	18,5
Half cross front	16	16,25	16,5	16,75	17
Crown height	13,5	14	14,5	15	15,5
Armhole (armscye) girth	37	38	39	40	41
Shoulder length	12,2	12,6	13,1	13,4	13,8
Total length of arms	58	60	62	64	66
Arm girth	25	26	27	28	29
Wrist girth	15,75	16	16,25	16,5	16,75
Height from waist to knee	57	58	59	60	61
Body rise	25	25,5	26	26,5	27

Body measurements

When compiling a specification sheet, the designer must consider a certain number of length and width measurements of the body.

The lengths are calculated in this way: the back is measured from the eighth vertebra (the prominent bone which protrudes at the top of the spine at the nape of the neck). The reference point for the front is at the shoulder point, which is situated where the base of the neck intersects the shoulder line. From these points several measurements can be established: chest height, from waist to chest, from waist to hip, from waist to knee, from waist to floor, from waist to back and from waist to front.

The widths, however, correspond to the measurements around the chest, waist and hips. The degree of shoulder slope will vary from one product to another. For example, a tee-shirt will vary from a jacket. However, this can be easily checked by using a protractor.

Manufacturers use standardised sizing which are generally classified in sizes from 8/16 in the UK (36–44 in Europe). A total knowledge of these measurements, which are listed in the chart above, is essential. You will notice that they increase by 4 cm per size. Therefore for a size 10/38, which is the reference size, the waist circumference is 66 cm, whereas it is 70 cm for a size 12/40.

Note that standard widths are established on a very variable basis which do not correspond to any garment. A design-er, therefore, must look at finished garments, and measure them, in order to have a good idea of the lengths and widths to give his/her samples. An idea of the desired volume for the garments will also need to be developed at this point.

So that the proportions and balance of the original model are respected, all the measurements corresponding to the different sizes, are carefully transferred onto the pattern (see p.156). Larger size models, those bigger than size 16/44, will require a new set of measurements and a new pattern. This is the same for the smaller sizes, which can either use children's sizing, or become a custom-made order.

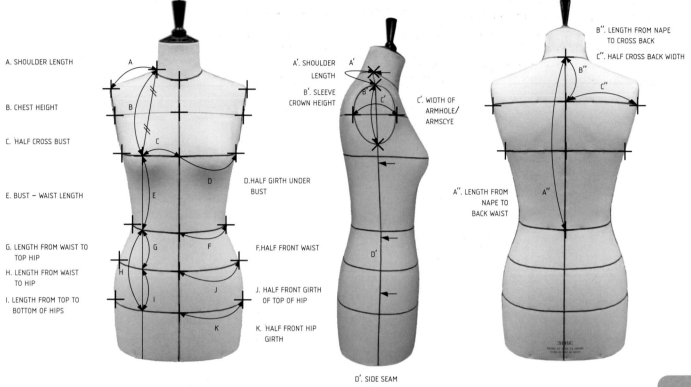

A. SHOULDER LENGTH

B. CHEST HEIGHT

C. HALF CROSS BUST

E. BUST – WAIST LENGTH

G. LENGTH FROM WAIST TO
   TOP HIP

H. LENGTH FROM WAIST
   TO HIP

I. LENGTH FROM TOP TO
   BOTTOM OF HIPS

D. HALF GIRTH UNDER
   BUST

F. HALF FRONT WAIST

J. HALF FRONT GIRTH
   OF TOP OF HIP

K. HALF FRONT HIP
   GIRTH

A'. SHOULDER
    LENGTH

B'. SLEEVE
    CROWN HEIGHT

C'. WIDTH OF
    ARMHOLE/
    ARMSCYE

D'. SIDE SEAM

B". LENGTH FROM NAPE
    TO CROSS BACK

C". HALF CROSS BACK WIDTH

A". LENGTH FROM
    NAPE TO
    BACK WAIST

Female dress-form size 10/38, with the principal lines needed for making a garment.

Dress form measurements

The dress form is an essential piece of studio equipment with measurements which correspond to the standard size of a female body, in this case. This three-dimensional representation of the female form serves as the link between the fashion illustration, the flat drawing, the human body and the garment. It is a useful aid in evaluating the garment and making the *toiles*.

In order to visualise the different parts of the body, measurement lines are positioned onto the dress form using a narrow black tape. These lines correspond to the reference points found on the fashion illustration (see p.147) and to the lines traced onto the pattern (see pp. 156–7). Three vertical axes symbolise the 'centre front', the 'centre back' and the sides. The front is 2 cm bigger than the back. The line on the side is always shifted 1 cm towards the back so that the seams do not appear on the front of the garment.

Perpendicular to these axes, the horizontal lines on the widest part of the back, chest, hips and waist allow the different garment pieces to be connected and balanced. The 'cut' then encourages a natural fall to the fabric. It is important to visualise these location marks on the body and take into consideration the need to move and breath easily. A garment can seem balanced on a dress form but, in reality, can be another matter – so adjustments might need to be made. When one designs a garment, it is important to try and visualise the piece in three-dimensions by imagining the volumes and proportions and reinterpreting them through his/her illustration.

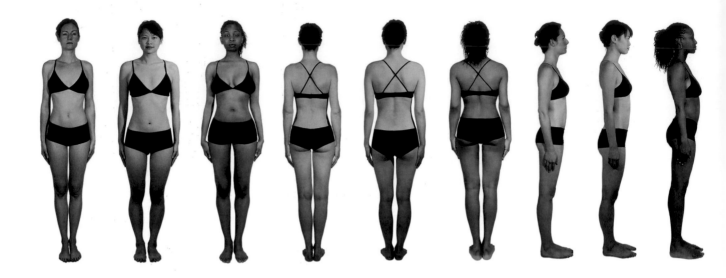

Morphology types

Body shapes vary according to the different regions of the world. Taming and overcoming nature in order to invent an environment to live in, man sculpted his own body. From the fashion world's perspective, it is important to consider these differences, which determine most of the constraints when designing products destined for particular markets.

Here, we consider three large groups – European, African and Asian – which we feel are representative of the morphology types most likely to be encountered. Naturally, there are distinctions amongst European body types. For example, between the Mediterranean and Nordic woman, whose hips and chests measurements vary. There are obvious differences between certain African tribes and likewise, between Japanese and Vietnamese people. Nevertheless, we feel that these three large categories sum up, appropriately, the diversity which results from the constant migrations and intermixing of these populations – a fact which has existed from the beginning of mankind.

Certain products have to be completely reconsidered according to the specific markets they address. Whether it be European, African or Asian, it is fundamental that the designer understands, and is capable of, creating garments which correspond to women from a particular morphology group.* Proportionally, one could say that, with the African body shape, the lower back region is more arched than it is with the European which, in turn, gives a shorter chest and a higher crotch in the sub-Saharan woman. On the other hand, in the Asian woman, the chest is longer, the legs shorter and the pelvis larger than in African and European women. This diversity continues ad infinitum and it has come full circle for, although it is the wish of certain women to make their silhouette appear somewhat unusual, the real world, the street and its 'natural' models are constant sources of inspiration for the fashion world and vice versa.

* *Certain items of clothing, such as the kimono, are the results of aesthetic research in relation to body morphology.

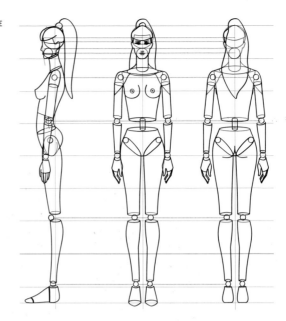

THE DEVELOPMENT OF A FASHION
ILLUSTRATION.

1. USING THE VOLUMES AND PROPORTIONS
FROM THE BASIC ILLUSTRATION, A LOP-SIDED
FIGURE IS DRAWN. THE SUPPORTING LEG MUST
BE POSITIONED IN THE AXIS WHICH GOES FROM
THE NECK TO THE FLOOR. THE HIGHEST PART
OF THE HIP IS IN THE EXTENSION OF THE SUP-
PORTING LEG. THE LINE OF THE SHOULDERS
SLOPE IN THE OPPOSITE DIRECTION TO THE
LINE OF THE PELVIS.

2. THE DRAWING IN FIG. 1 IS PLACED ON A
LIGHTBOX. A WHITE SHEET OF PAPER IS POSI-
TIONED OVER THE TOP OF IT AND THE OUTLINE
IS TRACED WITHOUT THE REFERENCE LINES.

3. THE GARMENT IS THEN DRAWN ONTO THE
OUTLINE.

4. THE ILLUSTRATION IS STYLISED BY USING
INK, FELT PEN, PENCIL ETC. TO ENHANCE THE
OUTLINE. THE ACCESSORIES, MAKE-UP AND
HAIRSTYLE ARE ADDED.

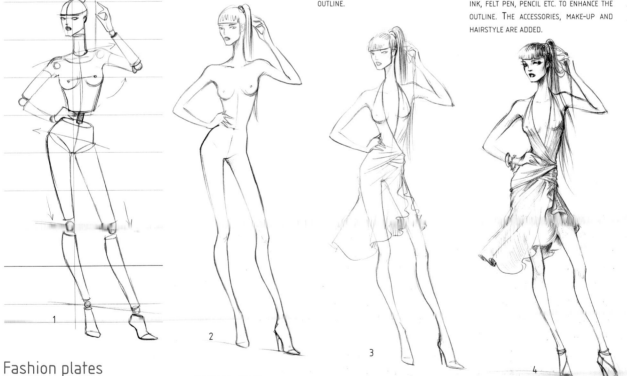

Fashion plates

These illustrations allow the designer to liberate his/ herself from the reality and constraints of specific body shapes. They do not represent a real female body as their androgynous appearance gives them idealised proportions. Gradually, the designer gives them an extremely stylised form which results in the finished fashion illustration.

These robotised illustrations have the advantage of providing reference points with which the designer can express his ideas for the 'flat' drawings and simulated volumes. It must be noted that the fashion illustration is not an artistic piece of work, rather a work tool. It is also better if it remains as static as possible, so as to avoid any confusion in the interpretation of the design.

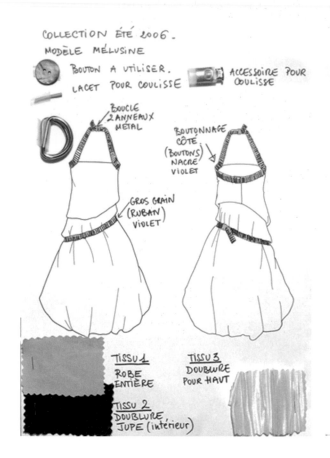

COLLECTION ÉTÉ 2006.
MODÈLE MÉLUSINE
BOUTON A UTILISER.
LACET POUR COULISSE   ACCESSOIRE POUR COULISSE

BOUCLE 2 ANNEAUX MÉTAL

BOUTONNAGE CÔTÉ (BOUTONS) NACRÉ VIOLET

GROS GRAIN (RUBAN) VIOLET

TISSU 1
ROBE ENTIÈRE

TISSU 3
DOUBLURE POUR HAUT

TISSU 2
DOUBLURE JUPE (intérieur)

		Réf.modèle prod : 3501/99	Réf.modèle studio : R58

Tissu 1

Tissu 3 (Intérieur haut)

Tissu 2 (Intérieur jupe)

Observations :

Tissu 1 :	Taffetas changeant DENIS (Extérieur)
Tissu 2 :	Doupion violet BELSOIE (Intérieur jupe)
Tissu 3 :	Lamé plissé CARLO VALLI (Intérieur haut)
Ceinture et bretelles :	Ruban gros grain violet

Observations du fabricant:

- Tissus fragiles : Ne pas repasser avec la presse à vapeur
- Attention au sens du tissu pour le taffetas changeant

Réf.modèle studio : R 58			Date : 20/05/2006	
Réf.modèle prod .: 3501/99			Fabricant : CHIC COUTURE	
Fournisseur	Réf.Tissu	Coloris	Laize	Composition
BELSOIE	réf.prod.: BE 350 Doupion	Violet	140 cm	100 % Soie
DENIS	réf.prod.: DE 628 Taffetas	Vert pâle	150 cm	51 % Soie 49 % Acétate
CARLO VALLI	réf.prod.: CV 732 Lamé plissé	Or pâle	140 cm	51 % Soie 49 % Polyester

Fournitures	Fournisseur	réf	Qté	Emplacement
Zip	YKK		1	
Ruban	Galonnade		2 m	
Griffe	Léon Weil	n°863/C	1	
Crochet	Léon Weil	n°45/A	1	
Boucle	Léon Weil	n°37	4	

A FLAT DRAWING OF A SPEC SHEET DESTINED FOR THE WORKROOM. IT SHOWS OUR MODEL OF THE DRESS MÉSULINE WHICH IS PRESENTED IN THE FINISHED ILLUSTRATION ON P. 97.

CONTRARY TO THE WORKROOM SPEC SHEET, WHICH GIVES ALL THE INSTRUCTIONS NECESSARY FOR THE PROTOTYPE'S MANUFACTURE, THE PRODUCTION SPEC SHEET HAS MORE DETAILED INFORMATION CONCERNING FABRIC QUANTITIES AND TRIMMINGS REQUIRED FOR SERIES PRODUCTION.

The 'flat' drawings, which accompany the fashion illustration, are stylised in the general spirit of the project. For example, if the project is about Pop Art, then one can opt for flat drawings which emulate the graphics and style of the superheroes used in American cartoons with a graphic feel close to that of the Pop artist Roy Lichtenstein.

When the technical drawing, or spec, goes to the workroom, it will be accompanied by instructions concerning the fabrics and trimmings for the pattern cutter. However, when these working drawings are destined for the production department, they are very rigorous and much more precise for the modeller needs as much information as possible about the garment. For example, symbols which indicate the position of stitches and other essential details, as well as the all important measurements, however, there will be certain ones which are only given as an approximation. This is because too many restrictions will hamper the modeller, inhibiting his or her creative input regarding volumes etc.

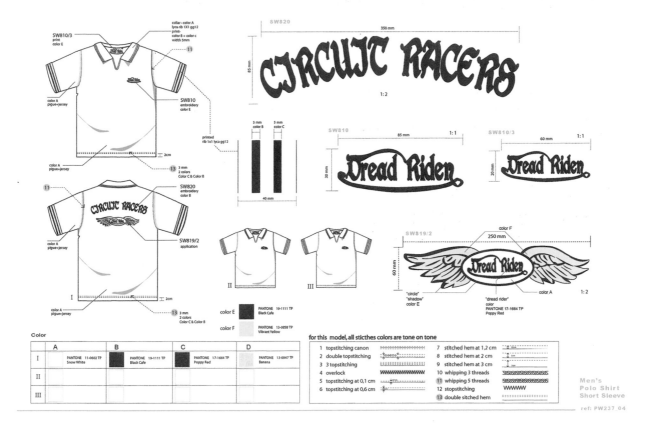

FLAT DRAWINGS FOR OUT-SOURCED PRODUCTION. THE SHEET IS ACCOMPANIED WITH ALL THE PANTONE REFERENCES FOR THE PRINTING, AND THE RELEVANT INSTRUCTIONS FOR THE TYPES OF STITCHES, POSITIONS OF MOTIFS AND TECHNIQUES USED (EMBROIDERED OR APPLIQUÉ).

The production spec sheets include a sketch, and all the instructions concerning the fabric (reference, weight, composition), manufacturing details, necessary trimmings (shoulder pads, buttons, zips, cloth, lining etc.).

So that a particular detail can be easily understood, the designer might draw a close-up of the product, or present the same detail from different angles. For example, the drawing of a pair of trousers might show them with the flies closed, and then a close-up of them open, to explain the finish.

Some technical drawings are so precise that they can be simulated as a working method, such as for knitwear where the diagrams indicate the manufacturing process and stitch textures.

A technical drawing must be explicit and give exact instructions. If in doubt, it is best to ask the atelier or supplier which material constraints should be considered and which essential instructions should feature.

It is important to be aware of the machines and tools to be used in the manufacturing process as the technique can vary according to which factory equipment is used.

For the production of a prototype garment, such as the dress made by the Lutz brand (pp.144–5), certain decisions will be made by the design consultants at the factory.

In the case of out-sourced manufacturing, such as with the polo shirt above, the spec sheets are very detailed as they will be used to make the prototype, which the designer will then confirm before launching it into large series production.

At the end of this chapter there is an example of an original construction technique showing how to easily make flat garment drawings.

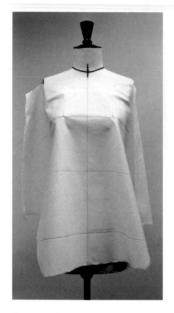

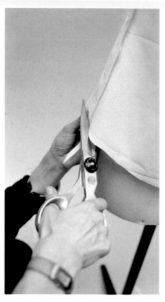

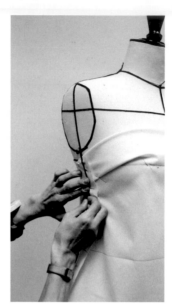

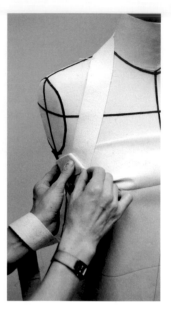

THE *TOILISTE* BEGINS BY PINNING THE *TOILE* ONTO THE DRESS FORM MAKING SURE THAT THE CENTRE FRONT GRAIN LINE (ALREADY TRACED ONTO THE *TOILE*) COINCIDES WITH THE CENTRE FRONT LINE ON THE DRESS FORM. THEN PIN THE MOST PROMINENT PART, IN THIS CASE THE BUST, ENSURING THE OTHER LOCATION MARKS COINCIDE.

SCISSORS ARE USED TO SNIP OFF ANY EXCESS FABRIC ON THE *TOILE*.

ANY EXCESS MATERIAL CAN BE INCORPORATED INTO A DART ON THE BUST.

THE SHOULDER STRAP IS PLACED IN SUCH A WAY THAT IT RESEMBLES A HALTER NECK AND AGAIN THE EXCESS FABRIC IS REABSORBED INTO A PLEAT.

Using the technical drawing supplied by the designer, the *toiliste* makes the prototype. There are two main ways of developing a garment shape: flat pattern-drafting or draping on a dress form.

Flat pattern-drafting consists of precision tracing, two-dimensionally, the different pieces which make up the garment. They are then cut and assembled three-dimensionally.

Draping involves fitting a *toile* fabric directly onto the dress form.

We have chosen the draping technique for our Mélusine example as it is the most appropriate method for the cut of the shape and the natural fall of the material – giving a lively and stylish aspect to the garment.

Draping is difficult to master and a highly regarded skill therefore it is important not to obscure the fabric whilst researching the garment shape. Someone with a practised eye, and who is familiar with fabrics, will derive great pleasure from draping a shape on a dress form and will obtain a better result than a modeller who has not yet mastered this art. We consider it a mistake to start one's apprenticeship by flat pattern-drafting as it can be somewhat approximate, rigid and limiting for the *toiliste*. Besides there are certain shapes which would be impossible to make without draping them first.

Before starting the process, the modeller irons the *toile* to remove any

finishes which might be on the fabric. By mastering this technique from the outset, sharp, precise results can be obtained.

Then, using a propelling pencil with a fine lead (0.3) and quite hard (H), trace the straight grain and the crosswise grain onto the fabric. These will assist in assembling the different pieces in order for the balance of the garment to hang straight. The straight grain coincides with the centre front line, the crosswise grain with the chest, waist and hip lines. The squares of this grid must always line up exactly in the middle of the side seams.

When fabric is used on the bias (to create drapes and flares or, for collars

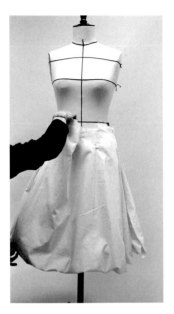 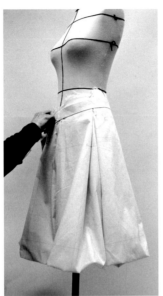 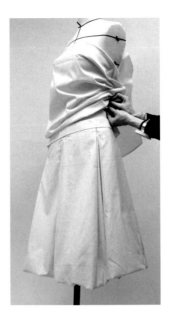 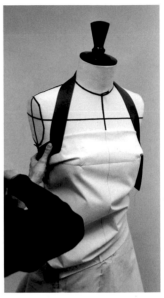

After having taken the top part of the *toile* off, the toiliste takes care of the skirt volume. Pleats are positioned around the waist.

Positioning an asymmetric waistband onto the skirt.

Once the skirt is finished, the *toiliste* replaces the top to make up the dress.

To give a more finished look, the *toile*'s shoulder strap is replaced by a piece of grosgrain fabric planned for the finished garment.

and belts where more stretch is required), the straight grain is at 45° to the centre front line, and to the waist line. The *toiliste* rotates the fabric 45° then traces the new waist, centre front and cross grain lines onto the *toile* to coincide with those on the dress form.

The notion of balance is crucial to the draping of standard designs and demands regular practice to understand and master it. The modeller begins by pinning or taping the *toile* in the centre front of the dress form (the garment's axes of reference being the centre front and waistline).

Volumes are achieved by working with folds, pleats, gathers etc. However, the natural fall of the fabric must be considered otherwise the garment will end up looking tortured and fall badly. Being able to master the rotations and swings of a fabric will result in a well-cut garment and, therefore, the directions of the grain lines and bias must be taken into account for each piece.

The tools used for draping consist of pins, tape, tape measure, scissors, pencil and tailor's chalk. To give the garment some volume, the excess is snipped off using the scissors and different coloured tape, either adhesive or ribbon, is used on the dress form to show the position of the shoulder straps and cutting lines. The folds, pleats, tucks and notches are marked using a pencil. (The notches are very useful when piecing together the different sections of the garment.) Pins are placed at regular intervals from the top to the bottom, slightly slanting to avoid any injury when removing.

Once the piece has been completely pinned and the *toiliste* is happy with the result, he/she uses a needlepoint tracing wheel along all the lines. These small holes will assist in the adjustment of the garment once it is removed from the dress form. The pins are carefully removed from each piece. Before removing the *toile*, the *toiliste* checks that there are no areas where he/she has forgotten to mark a seam due to being hidden by the pinned fabric.

Toïle making: truing

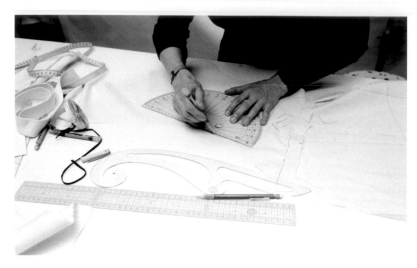

The lines are retraced onto the *toïle* using a protractor and coloured pen.

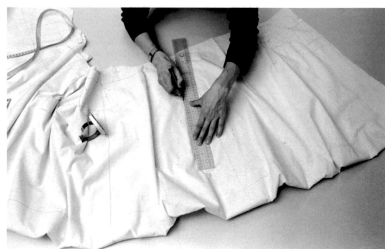

One after the other, the pins are removed from the pleats then the direction, edges and pleats are marked using a coloured pen and Japanese ruler.

When the garment is symmetrical, only one side of the *toïle* is worked on (the right side), however, if it is asymmetrical the entire model is worked, as in our example. Once the *toïle* has been removed from the dress form, all the pieces are ironed before laying them flat on the cutting table.

The different pieces of the *toïle* are placed onto the table with the back and the front, side by side (the centre backs and fronts parallel). The remaining pieces which make up the pattern are then positioned resembling a puzzle.

Adjustments consist of measuring and re-establishing the lines in relation to the grain line; checking the balance points of the pieces; verifying the arm-holes and necklines; the sides and hems, as well as the crotch in the case of a pair of trousers. The pleats, darts and folds are measured. The length of the darts, in the front, must not exceed 9 cm from the waist on the skirt part, however, those on the back can be up to 12 cm long.

The notches are checked and adjusted in relation to each other, if necessary.

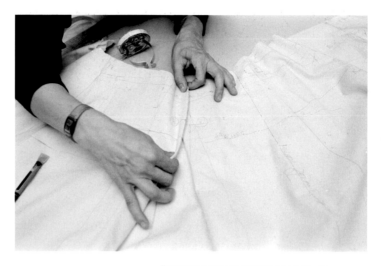

THE MEASUREMENTS ARE CHECKED WITH A TAPE MEASURE.

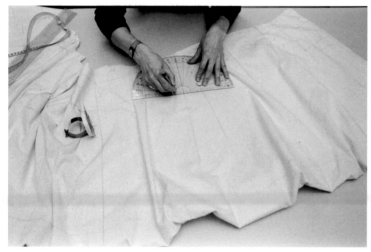

PLACING A LOCATION POINT WITH THE AID OF A PROTRACTOR INDI-
CATES WHERE THE PLEAT WILL BE SEWN.

When assembling the front and the back, it is important they do not form folds at the armholes, collar, waist and hem of the garment. To avoid this, the pieces must be lined up at right angles and so that natural curves are obtained, they must be pointing in the axis of these lines.

The height, length and widths are measured and eventually adjusted to the desired size. It is also important to ensure that the front and the back are always 2 cm different.

A coloured pen is used to mark precisely, clearly and neatly all the corrections that have been marked on the *toile*.

Finally, the seam allowances need to be made large enough for any correction, if necessary, during the fittings.

After finishing the adjustments the *toiliste* replaces the *toile* onto the dress form so that the fall can be verified and, if the work has been carried out carefully, the *toile* will give a precise idea of the final garment.

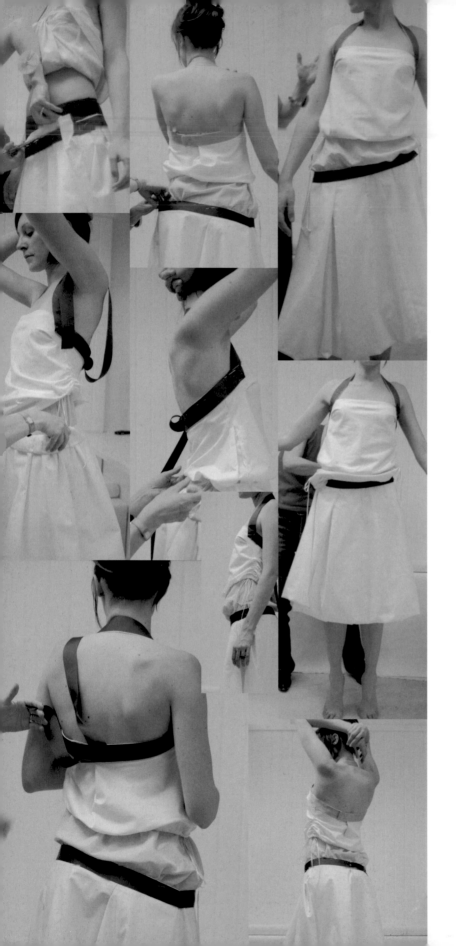

Toile making: fitting

The different fittings are carried out in front of the designer, the atelier manager and the toiliste with the aim of refining the garment on a real model. Depending on the difficulty of the garment, the number of fittings and adjustments, before the pattern-making stage, can be more than the two we are showing here.

First fitting

The fitting which happens after the first adjustment shows whether the designer's sketches have been adhered to in relation to the proportions, lines and style. It is also the first time that the designer and the modeller will have collaborated. As we have already seen, the first reaction to the garment and the fall of the fabric can prompt further research, that is why it is important to choose, in the first place, the materials best adapted to the garment. At this point, the person in charge of fabrics proposes the other samples which have been ordered as a sample length from the fabric supplier. The latter will be folded, or rolled, and hung on a clothes rack in the atelier.

   The unlined garment is not sewn, but tacked (using large stitches to hold the seams together, which are easy to undo if necessary) or simply pinned. It is essential, at this stage, that the modeller anticipates the seam allowances, making them big enough for any eventual alterations. Tailor's chalk, or tape, is used to mark any alteration lines directly onto the garment. In spite of their practical aspect, waxy chalks which disappear when ironed, are not advisable as they can leave marks on delicate fabrics.

Second fitting

the second fitting, before the pattern-making stage, the sample is cut from the sample length fabric that the designer has chosen to make the prototype sample in.

The garment is assembled, using large stitches, with its lining. It looks like the finished item but the details will be added later. In order to make it easier, or modify its overall look if necessary, allowances need to be taken into account, as with the first fitting. The seams are indicated by a tacked thread which allows the modeller to easily find the original lines. However, it is important to be aware that with certain materials, such as silk and leather, the tacked seams will leave an impression.

The prototype sample will not be able to be altered after the fitting and so will be abandoned and a new one made. These test pieces, however, will be able to be sold on in the press sales which are held after the fashion show.

Final fitting

This fitting is where the final alterations are made and is used particularly with haute couture items. The sample is adjusted on the model who is going to wear it at the fashion show, or on the client, in the case of an order. Great care is taken with this sample in particular, for it is the finished article and a unique garment which is regarded as a work of art. The finishing touches and ironing can take hours. The collars, cuffs and hemlines must not be crushed so they are rolled to keep the fullness of the fabric. The garment is entirely supported by reinforcing materials (linings, interlinings, interfacings, shoulder pads etc.) and held by tacking threads which are pulled out once the sample is finished.

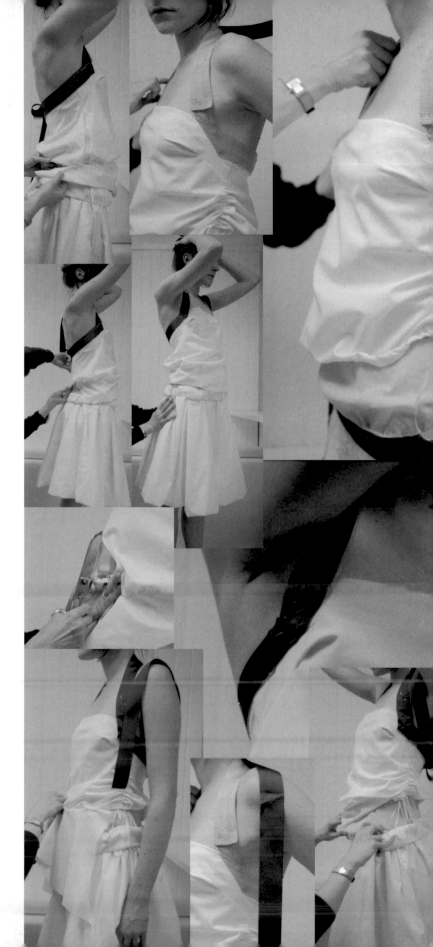

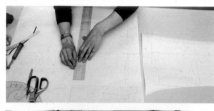

THE MEASUREMENTS ARE MADE USING A PERSPEX RULER AGAINST A SET SQUARE.

THE ARMHOLES AND DIFFERENT CURVES ARE MADE USING A FRENCH CURVE.

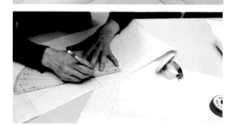

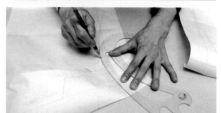

THE ANGLE OF THE SLOPE FOR CERTAIN LINES, SUCH AS THE SHOULDERS, IS MADE USING A PROTRACTOR.

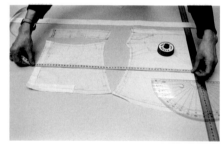

THE PATTERN CUTTER MAKES SURE THE CENTRE FRONT AND CENTRE BACK LINES ARE PARALLEL BEFORE CHECKING THE PATTERN. THE PIECES ARE PLACED NEXT TO EACH OTHER IN THE ORDER OF ASSEMBLY.

To make a pattern, a flat impression is produced of all the corrected *toile* pieces which will eventually go to make up the finished garment. Using a pattern tracing wheel, the pieces are traced onto a sheet of flexible card for woven fabrics, or rigid card for leather. These pieces then become known as the pattern.

Even in the case of an asymmetric item, these are then traced out as a complete shape, for in industry the cut is always done with the fabric open and not folded (see p.161). The centre front, centre back and waist are marked on the pattern. These axes allow the item to be gradated in four different sizes: 8(36), 12(40), 14(42), 16(44). Smaller or larger than those and a new prototype will need to be made.

The modeller uses different coloured marker pens to distinguish the different tracing lines – black for the main fabric, red for the linings, and green for fusible interfacings. Instructions are written on the right side of the pattern, which will then be placed face up onto the fabric for tracing.

The pattern cutter then uses a pair of compasses to transfer the outline of the garment taking into account the seam allowances: 1cm generally for classic seams, 0.5 cm for necklines and cuffs and 3 cm for a single-folded hemline. These measurements can, of course, vary depending on the machines and tools used during the assembling.

THE MODELLER USES PATTERN NOTCHERS TO MARK THE PATTERN.

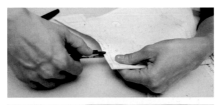

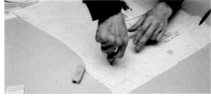

THE END OF A DART IS MARKED USING AN AWL.....

....THE DIRECTION OF A PLEAT IS MARKED BY A PATTERN TRACING WHEEL.

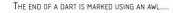

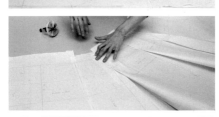

THE PATTERN CUTTER ADJUSTS THE DIFFERENT PIECES OF THE PATTERN OF A PLEATED SKIRT BEFORE RETRACING THE WAISTLINE.

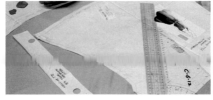

THE GARMENT SKETCH, NAME, REFERENCE, AND PATTERN SIZE ARE MARKED ON THE BACK PATTERN PIECE.

The sewing notches will indicate the armholes, hemlines, waist and position of inlays and zip fastenings etc. Every detail is meticulously marked.

The card is perforated in the places which correspond to the limit of the pins and the pocket outlines so that they can be marked onto the fabric for the cut. This last operation is essential when assembling mass-produced items.

Finally, special templates are made for pockets, collars and buttonholes – the curves, angles, directions and widths all need to be precisely detailed. These templates include the detail of the pattern piece concerned, without the seams. The quantity of pieces which make up the pattern, and their reference numbers are marked on the reverse of each piece. Information such as the season, the collection, name of item, reference, size and accompanying sketch are also recorded here.

The entire pattern is carefully laid out with the smaller pieces fitting in between the larger pieces of the front and back. As they are placed back to front on the fabric, this arrangement leaves all the information and lexicon easily visible. Once made, all the pieces are attached together either using tape, or by a pattern hook passed through a perforated hole in the cards.

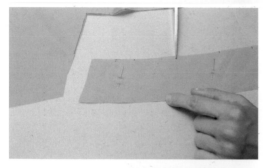

THE CUTTER USES SHEARS TO CUT A NOTCH IN THE FABRIC ACCORDING TO THE PATTERN INSTRUCTIONS.

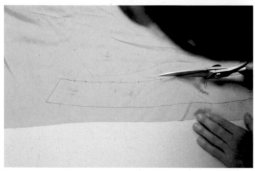

THE PIECES ARE CUT FOLLOWING THE LINE OF THE TAILOR'S CHALK. ONE HAND CUTS WHILST THE OTHER HOLDS THE FABRIC FLAT ON THE CUTTING TABLE.

In the workroom

The fabric, which has been rolled up on its right side, is unrolled and the different pattern pieces are positioned so as to have the least amount of material waste as possible. This positioning defines the lay plan which will be followed for the mass-production of the garments whilst the linings and supporting fabrics have their own lay plans. All these plans are attached to the item's technical file.

The cutter must take into account fabric's direction when placing the pattern pieces. They must be positioned in the straight grain line, in one direction or another, depending on the nature of the material – for example, the nap of a velvet fabric looks different depending on the direction, as is also the case with printed fabrics. The notches will help indicate the balance and direction of the pattern.

To make a prototype sample, the cutter traces the outline of the pattern pieces onto the fabric using tailor's chalk, marks the notches and the pockets in pencil. For greater precision and to gain time, a symmetrical item can be folded in two, face to face, and cut with shears exclusively reserved for this process (although, as already mentioned, this does not apply to industry).

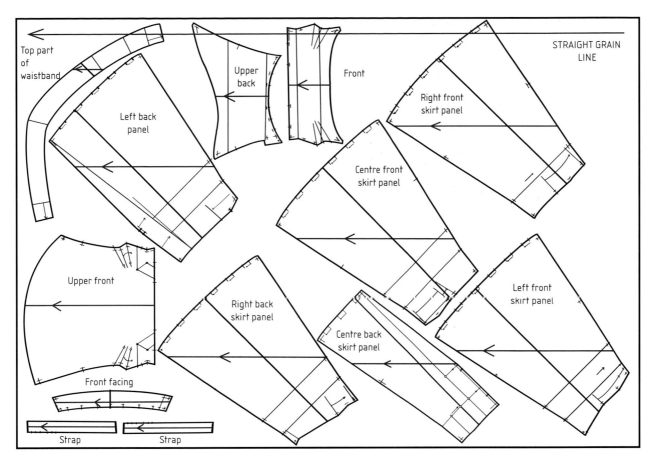

Top part of waistband

Upper back

Front

STRAIGHT GRAIN LINE

Left back panel

Right front skirt panel

Centre front skirt panel

Upper front

Right back skirt panel

Centre back skirt panel

Left front skirt panel

Front facing

Strap

Strap

CUTTING PLAN SHOWING THE POSITIONING OF THE PATTERN PIECES ON THE FABRIC.

In industry

For mass-produced items, the outlines of all the items are traced onto pattern paper (similar to, but thinner than, tracing paper). This is then placed onto the opened-out fabric.

From a large, horizontal fabric roll, the pattern-cutter and an assistant unroll the necessary lengths of fabric onto the cutting table. There needs to be sufficient to make a determined number of samples. He places as many layers of fabric, on top of each other, as there are items to be cut – this makes up what is known as a 'mattress' which can, in turn, be made up of different coloured fabrics, if necessary.

The marking of notches, darts, pockets and buttonholes is done with a heated drill, or laser. And electric shears, with circular or vertical blades, are used to cut through the layers of fabric.

Some factories are equipped with laser-cutting material. Certain equipment manufacturers, such as Gerber or Lectra, propose tracing software programmes and fully-automated cutting equipment to the industry.

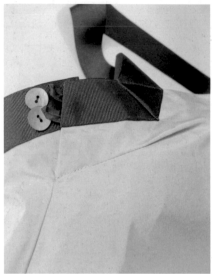

A DETAIL OF THE LEFT SIDE SEAM AT THE TOP OF THE DRESS: TWO LOOPED BUTTONHOLES, WITH BUTTONS, PLACED ON A GROSGRAIN RIBBON. THE EXCESS FABRIC ON THE BUST IS TAKEN UP BY A DART WHICH ENDS IN A SMALL FOLD. IT IS NOT FLATTENED OUT WITH IRONING BUT LEFT TO BOUNCE BACK.

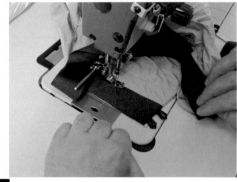

THE MACHINIST BEGINS BY SEWING THE WAISTBAND BY HAND. IT IS FIXED ONTO THE DRESS USING A SEWING MACHINE AND STRAIGHT STITCH.

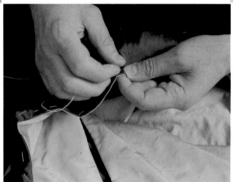

The sample machinist

This is the person, in an atelier, who very carefully assembles the prototype pieces. It is at this stage that any problem with the pattern are flagged up and corrected for the production. The machinist works in close collaboration with the *toiliste* who made the sample, at this point, as well as the pattern-making stage. For a skilled sample machinist understands cutting and pattern-making. He, or she, will advise the *toiliste* on the best techniques for making the details, which are generally the most simple and aesthetic. It is with this knowledge that the garment becomes finished. For example, he, or she, will be able to correct certain errors, or hide an excess of material into a seam.

The seams can be pressed open or pressed to one side and top-stitched. Top-stitched seams are usually used on garments which require strengthening, in the case of sportswear, casual wear, children's wear and work clothes. Certain materials, such as leather, will automatically require top-stitching as do details such as flat pockets, which can only be fixed to a garment by this technique. The sample machinist adjusts the length of the top-stitch and can change the colour of the thread to give it the appearance of a saddle stitch.

In the *haute couture* world, all the

finishing details are carried out by hand. Bias cutting and pleat work demand particular care – reminiscent of the dresses of Madame Grès and Madelaine Vionnet – and can only successfully be done by hand.

The final stage of this process is the ironing which helps with the overall fall and finish of the item. Certain items require hours of ironing, in particular those with sleeves and suit collars etc.

The industrial machinist

In industry, the machinist is a specialised craftsman who deals with the rendering and assembling of the piece, without correcting any eventual mistakes. This is why the corrections identified by the sample machinist must, without fail, be transferred onto the pattern by the *toiliste* (or by the design consultants).

A range of equipment is used depending on the different requirements. For example, when assembling seams, a flat sewing machine is used, shirts are made using a machine which specialises in American or 'felled' seams, leather is worked using double or triple cams, and a finishing technique used for knitwear, which over-locks and assembles the garment in one operation, blind hemming on scarves etc.

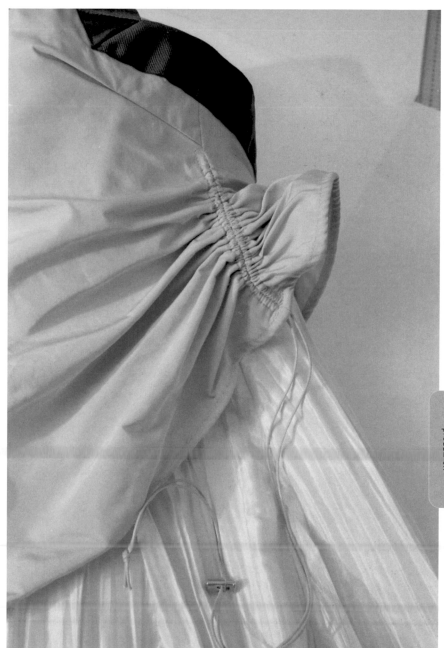

DETAILS OF THE LEFT SIDE SEAM AT THE TOP OF THE DRESS: A DRAWSTRING MAKES A SERIES OF GATHERS. THE HEMLINE IS FOLDED UP TWICE

Flat drawing for a straight skirt

Flat drawings are constructed on a reduced scale, which must be defined before the tracing is started. We have used measurements in this example which correspond to a size 10(38) in reality.

Each product needs to be based on real garment measurements so do not be tempted to do it freehand!

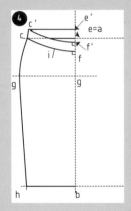

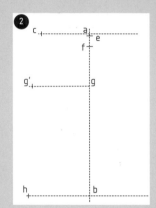

Trace the depth of the back waist *(ae)*. Sometimes this depth can be confused with the waistline as in our example *(e = a)*.

Trace the depth of the front waist *(af)*.

On the right, place point g which corresponds to the height of the hips. This is situated at 19-20 cm from point a in a size 10 (38).

Trace a ¼ circumference of the hips *(gg')* which is equal to 92 divided by 4 (fitting tightly on the dress form) therefore 23 cm more or less for a size 10 (38).

Trace half the hem width *(bh)*.

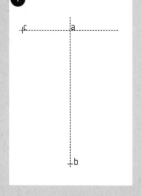

Trace the height of the waistband *(cc')*, *(ff')*, *(ee')*.

Join the points f and c, c and g', g' and h, h' and b, to obtain the line of half of the front of the skirt. Then join points *e'* and *c'*, *f'* and *c'* to trace the waistband.

Place the starting point for the dart *(i)*. The darts are placed a 6-7 cm from the centre front under the waistline *(fc)* – the lengths of which must not exceed 9 cm in the front.

If there is a secondary dart, put it halfway between the first dart(i) and the side seam of the skirt *(c)* for a classic style.

Draw the top stitching, darts, fastenings and all the other details which figure on your model.

Trace the other half of the skirt, taking the centre front line as your symmetry axis *(fb)*

From the front impression, trace the back placing a seam in the centre back, if necessary. Symbolise the zip by a zig-zag.

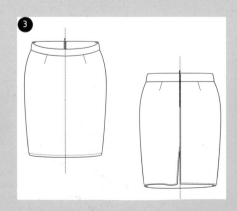

Trace the skirt length *(ab)*.

Trace half the circumference of the front waist (ac), which is equal to 66 cm divided by 4, therefore 16, 5 cm, for a size 10 (38). To make it look better, you can slightly reduce this measurement.

For a low waist, the waist is placed 9 cm below the waistline. Consequently, the half circumference of the front waist *(ac)* will vary.

> Don't forget the skirt openings, using zips or buttons. If a zip is used on the side, place it on the left.

Flat drawing of a pair of straight-legged trousers

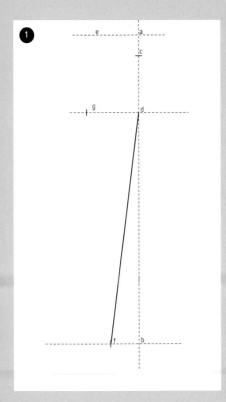

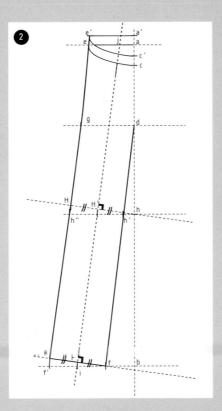

Trace the lines perpendicular to line *(ij)* from point *h'* , for the knee line and point *(f)* for the trouser bottom. Plot points H,H', F and F' on these lines so that *(h', H')* = (H' H) for the knee line, and *(f F')= (F'F)* for the bottom. These measurements will vary depending on the shape of the trousers.

Join points F, H, *g, e,* and *c* to trace half the trouser front. Plot points *a', c'* and *e'*. Join points *a'* and *e', e* and *c*, and finally *a* and *e* to determine the height of the waistband.

Place the dart, if there is one, under the waistline *(ec)*. This falls on the straight grain line *(ij)*.

Trace the total height *(ab)* (= 110 cm for example), the depth of the front of the waist (ac) , the height of the rise (cd) (more or less 25 cm) and the ¼ circumference of the waist (ae).

Plot point *(d)* on the line (ab) , this determines the height *(cd)* of the rise. Then trace the line (dg), perpendicular to the line (ab). This corresponds to ¼ circumference of the pelvis. (NB: This is called the hip measurement even if, in reality, it is situated below the hips.)

Finally, trace half the spread of the legs (bf). Trouser legs are very spread out (approx. 40 cm). On your drawing, reduce this measurement to 20 cm to make it look better. Then divide this measurement by two as only half the drawing is traced.

Join the points *f* and *d*.

Plot point h on the line *(ab)*, this corresponds to the height of the knee. (ah) is equal to the length of the waist to the knee (60-60 cm.) On the drawing, plot point *h* halfway along the trouser length (at 55 cm, i.e. 110 divided by 2). This will make it look better.

From point *(h)*, trace a line perpendicular to line *(ab)*. This cuts *(fd)* at h'. Plot point *h''* so that *(h' h'')* equals the width of the knee. Extend *(bf)* and plot point *f* so that *(ff')* equals the width of the trouser bottom.

Plot point *i* in the middle of *(ff')* and point *i* in the middle of *(h'h'')*. Trace the line which passes through *i* and *i'* and place point *j* at the intersection of this line and that of line *(ae)*. This line corresponds to the straight grain line of the trousers. Here you can check the precision of your drawing : after having scaled it up to life-size, verify that point *j* is 6-7 cm from the centre front of a size 10 (38) pair of trousers.

> Do not forget to convert the measurements marked here to the scale of your drawing.

Flat drawing of a pair of straight-legged trousers

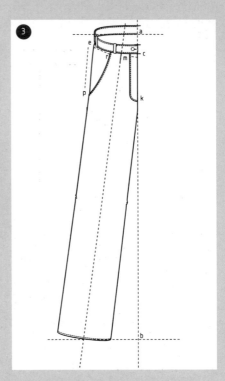

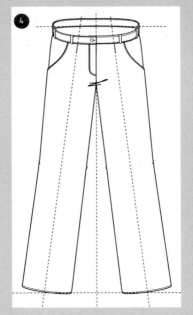

Trace the entire front of the pair of trousers, symmetrically. Using the impression of the front, trace off the back, with all the details, paying attention to crotch on the back which rises higher than the front. It is very important to include the profile as this shows the style of trouser i.e. straight, wide, flared etc.

Align the three drawings on the same reference points (waist, crotch, knee and bottom lines) to check that the heights all correspond.

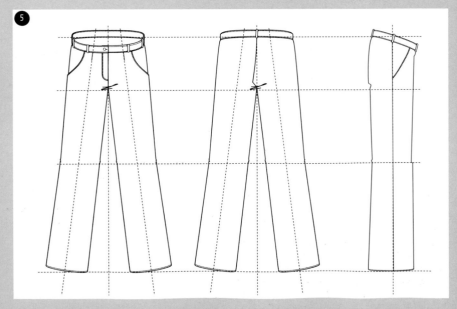

Now position the details. Trace the height of the fly opening *(ck)* , the width *(mc)*, the height of the pocket (ep), and opening *(er)*.

From point m trace a line parallel to *(ck)* which peters out to a round at point *k*. The flies will vary again depending on the style of the trousers. Finally, trace on the belt loops (normally, for each half front – one on the front, side and back) and all the other details by joining up the corresponding points.

Flat drawing for a long-sleeved tee-shirt

To begin trace half the front left body, then the sleeve.

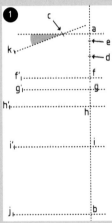

(kh') is equal to the height of the armhole (14-18 cm).

Join points e, c, k, f', g', h', i', j, b, and d, c to trace the outline of half the front.

Plot points c', e', d', so that (cc') = (dd') = (ee') = the height of the collar.

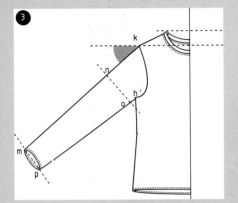

Trace line (ab) which corresponds to the entire length of the tee-shirt. Then trace a line perpendicular to (ab), passing through point, a and plot point c, which corresponds to the shoulder point on this perpendicular. Length (ac) is equal to the half-opened neckline.

Plot points d and e on the line ab, ad being equal to the depth of the front of the neck line. Plot points f, g, h, i, on (ab). The following lengths are then determined : shoulder point / cross chest ((af) = 10 cm), shoulder point/ cross bust ((ag) = 14 cm), shoulder point / chest ((ah) = 23 – 26 cm),

chest/waist ((hi) = 16-18 cm).

From these points , trace the perpendiculars onto the line ab, and plot points f', g', h', i', and j so that (ff') is equal to the front top half-chest , (gg') to the lower front half-bust,(hh') to the front half-chest, (ii') to a quarter circumference of the waist and (bj) to the half-width of the bottom of the shirt.

From the neck line, point c, use a protractor to trace the shoulder line taking into account the angle (in our example it is 20°). On this shoulder line, plot point k ; (ck) is equal to the shoulder length (= 10-12 cm).

Using a lightbox, from the centre front line trace the other side symmetrically. This will give you the entire tee-shirt. Use the front impression to trace the back modifying the cross back and the neckline.

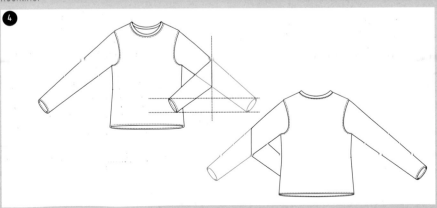

From point k which corresponds to the shoulder limit, use a protractor to trace the line above the sleeve taking into account the angle of the slope (about 30–35°). Plot point m at this juncture; (km) equals the sleeve's length (58–60 cm).

Plot point n on the line (km) ; (kn) being more or less 12 cm. From point n , trace the perpendicular (no), this equals the width of the arms. From point m, trace the perpendicular(mp), which equals the opening at the bottom of the sleeve. Join up points k, m, p, o, h' to obtain the line of the sleeve.

Do not forget to draw on the stitching, pockets and all the other details which figure on the model. The more the drawing is like the original, with the least amount of details, the more it will work.

Flat drawing for a shirt

The order of tracing for a shirt is as follows: front left half body, collar, button stand, other details, cuff and finally the back.

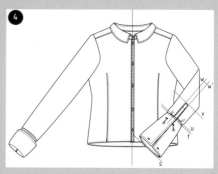

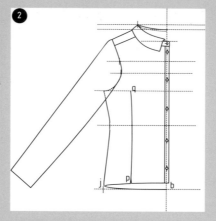

Trace the height of the cuff *(st)*, the height of the shirt stand *(uv)* and the width of the buttonhole stand *(ww')*

Fold one sleeve back so that the front and the back detail of the sleeve's cuff and opening figures on the same drawing. If the cuff is of a musketeer type, (like in our example), then consider drawing it folded and unfolded. Square off the buttonhole stand.

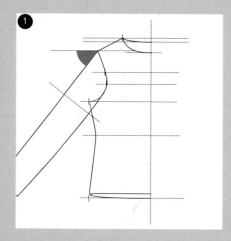

Trace on the button stand, indicating the direction of the buttonsholes.

The buttonhole at the base of the collar is always horizontal, whereas when they are on the stand, they are vertical. Place the buttonholes on the axis *(ab)* making sure they are symmetrical. Once this is determined, the width of the stand will become apparent.

Trace the length of the front dart *(pq)*, chest pockets and shoulder strips if there are any on your model. Every detail of the shirt must figure on the flat drawing with instructions concerning stitches and seams, in particular.

Using a lightbox, trace off symmetrically the centre front left.

When you trace the collar, consider lifting one side of it to show the assembly (stitches). Trace *(cl)*, the height of the collar and *(no)*, the fall of the collar. The overlap measurement *(em)* varies depending on the size of the buttons used. When tracing this, make sure that the buttons are placed in the centre front of the shirt. You must, therefore, take the measurement between point m and the axis *(ab)* . The height of the yoke *(kk')* depends on the type of shirt.

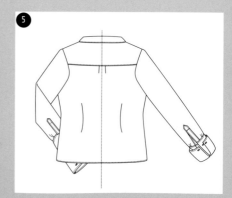

Use the same process as the tee-shirt to trace the front of a shirt. However, pay attention to the shoulder – sleeve angle (40–45°) which is more pronounced on a shirt. The shoulder angle, on the other hand, stays the same (20°). Trace the sleeve, without the cuff ,in the same manner as that of the tee-shirt.

(ab) = centre front, total length;
(ac) = neckline opening ;
(ad) = back neckline depth ;
(ae) = front neckline depth ;
(ff') = ½ cross front; *(gg')* = ½ cross chest
(hh') = ¼ chest circumference; *(ii')* = ¼ waist circumference;
(bj) = ½ bottom front width; *(ck)* = shoulder length;
(kx) = sleeve length (without the cuff);
(xx') = opening at bottom of sleeve;
(ww') = sleeve width.

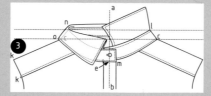

From the front impression, trace off the back. Think about modifying the yoke, the arm holes, the width between the shoulders and the pleat (for men, rounded, hollow or flat) or state with the model has gathers etc.

Flat drawing of a suit jacket

Use the same method as for the shirt, considering the collars, armholes and different details which are particular to this product.

Be careful not to take the impression of a tee-shirt, or shirt/blouse for each of these products have a completely different cut: the tee-shirt is knitwear, the shirt is a non-fitted product, like a dress, and a jacket is a tailored cut.

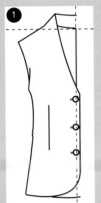

Body tracing

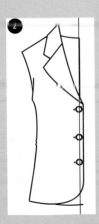

Collar tracing and its angle

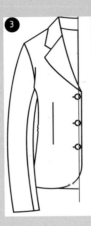

Sleeve tracing

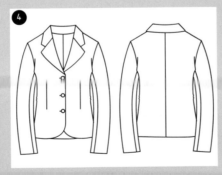

Flat drawing of the front and back of a straight suit jacket with three buttons and lined.

> You can also show the sleeves folded, as we have done in our example for the tee-shirt and shirt. This allows you to present the cuffs, front and back, on the same drawing, which is most important in the case of a shirt.

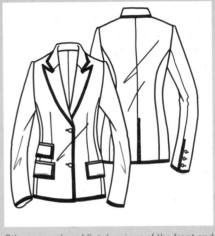

Other examples of flat drawings of the front and back of a straight suit jacket.

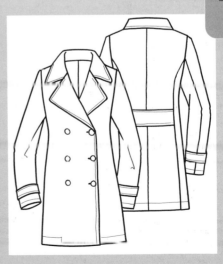

Examples of flat drawings of the front and back of a long reefer jacket.

Nowadays the fashion sector requires ever-increasing budgets to take care of the promotional and marketing campaigns of its brand images and product sales. A company's PR (public relations) department will organise a whole range of high-profile media events including fashion shows, product launch parties, and 'happenings' for boutique openings – an example of this being the opening night of Louis Vuitton's large department store on the Champs Elysées, in Paris with performance artist Vanessa Beecroft.

The organisation of a fashion show involves a large number of people: first of all, a producer, who is responsible for arranging the place and choreography of the show (either by himself or with the help of a choreographer); a press officer, who takes care of the invitations and press coverage. Eventually bookings will need to be made for the models and their entourage, which include hairdressers, make-up artists, dressers; a variety of technicians for sound mixing and lighting; security guards; caterers; artists and musicians and finally, all sorts of assistants will be recruited to coordinate such an occasion.

A veritable 'armada' is needed to ensure the successful promotion of a collection: merchandisers, who choose the commercial pieces which need to be incorporated into the show; PR companies or independent press officers; event organisers, publicity agents; fashion journalists, who work in collaboration with the show's producer; fashion editors, stylists, photographers, illustrators, interior decorators, graphic designers etc. To ensure maximum exposure, the media is courted as the fashion show (and its build-up) will be televised, in the press and on the Internet.

Today, it is the artistic directors, whose styles are synonymous with a particular brand image, who orchestrate these events. For example, John Galliano or Hedi Slimane for Dior, Karl Lagerfield for Chanel, Nicolas Ghesquière for Balenciaga, or Alber Elbaz for

Lanvin. The shop windows also contribute greatly to the fashion show's promotion, for it is often the artistic directors themselves who dress them, as in the case of Alber Elbaz for Lanvin.

Film festivals, such as Cannes, and Deauville, and the presentation of the Oscars, are also significant promotional platforms. It is here that the press office will solicit celebrities to wear clothes and accessories from a particular brand. In some cases, fashion stylists are employed to dress the stars which, in turn, contributes to the promotion of a fashion house. Finally, top-level sporting personalities can be sponsored by a particular brand – all of which adds to the high-profile exposure.

The key to successful promotion, however, lies in publicity campaigns with the press, advertising, radio and the increasingly thriving Internet. (Note that there are a number of sites and blogs dedicated to the fashion world, which are easily accessible and where information is updated daily.)

The press, which is generally, largely financed by publicity, makes an increasing effort to satisfy their advertisers by offering regular editorials.

Today, brands will call in specialised design collectives such as *Surface2 air Paris* or *Work in Progress* to help with promotion as they are able to target larger market sectors.

In this final chapter, we have chosen to illustrate the promotional aspects of a product by accentuating the fundamental role of the press office and PR department, as well as depict 'a fashion product' using a series of visual means. Therefore to represent our dress 'Mésuline', we have enlisted the help of illustrator, Antoine Kruk and photographer, Stéphan Shopferer.

We also explain the work of the fashion stylist and photographer, make-up artist and hairdresser then conclude, by going backstage at a fashion show.

It is the person in charge of public relations (PR) who is ultimately responsible for the brand's promotion, and that of its products. It can be someone who is incorporated in the brand's company, with the title of 'director of communications', or someone working in an independent PR company. The latter use showrooms where they present and promote different products and brands. Their role is to place a product into the market, impose its image on the public and make sure that the brand image is respected or redefined, if necessary, in close collaboration with the artistic director and merchandiser. They can also be the link between the company and any eventual partners in the case of a licence (where a designer works in conjunction with industry and royalties are involved).

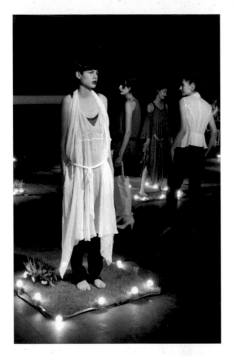

Presse release

This contains text concerning the presentation of the brand, designer, season's themes, as well as visuals (photographs/illustrations) showing the look. It is the stage where the fashion stylist and photographer establish a coherent iconography. The press release also includes descriptions of the items, list of retail outlets for the brand and finally a price list.

Events management

The PR is responsible for planning strategic publicity events such as product launches, shop/boutique openings, presentation of the collections, new lines and products, or even an event marking the presence of the brand in a new country (see Sourcing and sales representative's office). The main events which he, or she, organises are the launch parties and the fashion shows, as well as, all the arrangements concerning the place, the model castings (for the shows), the invitations, the press releases etc. He, or she, compiles an extensive list of contacts which include the press, art and theatre personalities, privileged clients, buyers from large department stores and buying houses.

Presse conferences

The PR, being the interface between the company and the media, is the person who organises the press conferences, press packs and exclusive interviews in order to establish a dialogue with the media.

Mail shots

Mail shots help to keep journalists informed of special events, such as press sales and open days which maintain good and positive professional relationships.

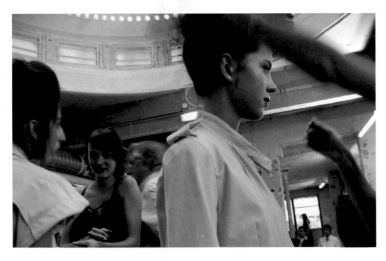

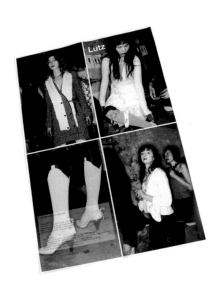

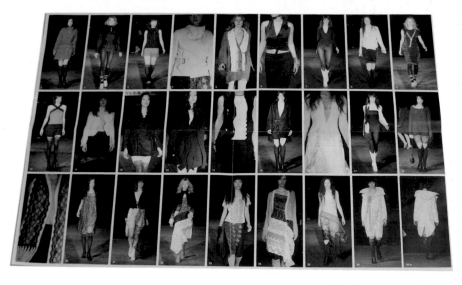

Lutz's autumn – winter 2006-2007 collection is presented as a brochure (both sides being shown here). The photos were taken during the fashion show.

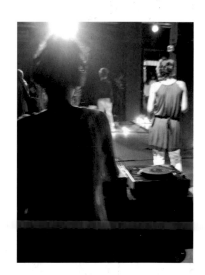

Advertising

The PR works in collaboration with advertising agencies in order to define and maximise the client's image choosing to advertise in, or on, the following formats: posters, hoardings, tabloid newspapers, specialist magazines and advertising slots either on the television, cinema, theatre or Internet etc.

Sourcing and sales representatives

The PR works in collaboration with advertising agencies in order to define and maximise the client's image choosing to advertise in, or on, the following formats: posters, hoardings, tabloid newspapers, specialist magazines and advertising slots either on the television, cinema, theatre or Internet etc.

In certain cases, the sales representative's office will intervene in the distribution strategy of a brand adapting its image to suit the market. This practice is common in the United States and Asia.

Sponsorship

This is where companies and/or institutions form partnerships with individuals or groups and work symbiotically for mutual publicity. The largest groups within the international textile industry have also associated themselves with sporting personalities and events - for example, Louis Vuitton and the 1998 World Cup with the famous football which was immortalised by the work of the sculptor Arman, or Nike with Michael Jordan or the Brazilian team. Another example, is the participation of the famous champagne house, Moet et Chandon, at the young designer's fashion shows which associates design with luxury.

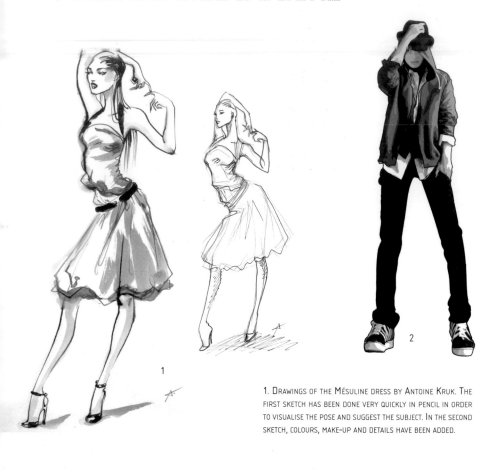

1. DRAWINGS OF THE MÉSULINE DRESS BY ANTOINE KRUK. THE FIRST SKETCH HAS BEEN DONE VERY QUICKLY IN PENCIL IN ORDER TO VISUALISE THE POSE AND SUGGEST THE SUBJECT. IN THE SECOND SKETCH, COLOURS, MAKE-UP AND DETAILS HAVE BEEN ADDED.

THIS ILLUSTRATION IS THE RESULT OF COMPUTER GRAPHICS COMBINED WITH A PHOTO-ENHANCING AND DRAWING PROGRAMME. AFTER HAVING DIGITALISED A PHOTO, THE ILLUSTRATOR REWORKS IT IN PHOTOSHOP (BACKGROUND REMOVED, FEET MADE LARGER AND LEGS THINNER). HE THEN USES THE SOFTWARE FILTERS – COMPARABLE, IN PRINCIPLE, TO THE FILTERS PLACED ON A CAMERA LENS – TO GIVE A GRAPHIC STYLE TO THE DRAWING. THE CHOSEN FILTER HERE SIMPLIFIES THE COLOUR ZONES, TRANSFORMING THE COLOUR GRADATIONS INTO FLAT AREAS OF COLOUR. THE RESULTING IMAGE IS IMPORTED INTO THE DRAWING SOFTWARE (ILLUSTRATOR) SO THAT THE OUTLINE OF THE SILHOUETTE CAN BE REDESIGNED.

The influence of digital technology

Today an illustrator is, more often than not, a graphic designer who has mastered new technologies and is able to create images by combining photography and illustration.

'Digital' styles appeared in the 1990s due to the evolution of graphic software and photo-enhancing, coupled with the rapidly expanding trends of street and sportswear. It would only be logical that these two market sectors, working to develop new materials from new technology, would look to a new generation of computer-literate illustrators to promote their brands.

Graphic designers have the advantage of being versatile: they can create a brand's visual image and develop it in a range of different media (posters, advertising booklets, on PVC hoardings etc.). This digital process has been facilitated by the advent of tools, such as the graphic tool boxes which replace the mouse with a 'digital crayon', the scanners which allow you to digitalise a drawing and the photographs which can be reworked on a computer. Notable exponents of this type of work are Annette Marie Pearcy, Stephane Goddard, Tatjana Jeremic, Autumn Whitehurst and Ling Chen.

These differ again from the technical drawing or the fashion illustration, both of which are necessary for the sample's manufacture, as they are the highest quality stylised sketches which are full of energy and generally abstracted.

It is essential to be able to capture a mood, or atmosphere, and include movement and life into the drawing. Concentrating on proportions, lines of direction and colours is more important than the construction details, in this case. An era is marked by its illustrations, graphics and moods. The illustrations of *La Belle Époque* made by Alphonse Mucha are emblematic of Art Nouveau at the beginning of the last century; in the 1920s it

was Erté's roses; in the 1950s it was the illustrations of René Gruau for Dior; in the 1970s, those of Antonio Lopez; in the 1980s, those of Thierry Perez and Tony Viramontes and in the 1990s, those of Mats Gustavson. However, during the 1960s photographers were more in vogue than illustrators, a trend which is endorsed by Antonioni's film *Blow Up*.

The beginning of the 21st century sees a strong return to illustration with, amongst others, Julie Verhoeven and Jean-Philippe Delhomme. A current example of this is with the concept-store Colette in Paris, which does not hesitate to use the talents of up-and-coming illustrators for the visuals in their shop windows.

The look

The choice of illustration used to present the 'look' of a collection is interesting as it can exaggerate certain characteristics, like a caricature does, and translate different stereotypes into one homogeneous whole. Normally, the look defines the image that one wants to portray to others enabling a succession of different identities.

It encompasses the comfort of a classic one, the confrontational spirit of others, such as punks, goths etc., or even shows a kind of social or professional 'belonging', as with a uniform.

The look presents typical silhouettes which have a dress-code belonging to a particularly urban 'tribe' – the way the garments are coordinated confirms the social group with which they identify themselves.

The phenomenon of urban tribes is perhaps a consequence of the disappearance of social divides and of supremacy, since the 1970s with the feminist movement and the androgynous model, incarnated by Jane Birkin – the eternal asexual adolescent. This supremacy is strongly confirmed with the masculine collections of Kenzo and Paul Smith, where the man is covered in floral patterns, and the work of Hedi Slimane for Dior's men's collection, where the models are young, slight men, barely out of their teens, contrasting dramatically with the muscle-bound men of the 1900s. Soft, supple fabrics and women's accessories have found a new 'niche'.

The study of 'looks' is a new sociological approach and it is a prerequisite for everyone to recognise and understand them in today's society. Equally, the look is a fashion phenomenon; it follows trends from the cosmic silhouettes of the 1960s with Courrèges, Pierre Cardin, Paco Rabanne, right up to the complex shapes which destruct the body, including the djellabas, tunics and bell-bottom 'hippie' trousers, the structured lines of the 1980s with Thierry Mugler, Claude Montana, and the minimalism of the 1990s with Prada, Helmut Lang, Jil Sander – to name but a few!

To show some current looks, we present here some extracts from the fashion illustrator, Antoine Kruk's book, *Shibuya Soul*. These different street attitudes have been taken from the trendy areas of Tokyo (Shibuya, Harajuku and Daikanyama).

1. CLUBBER
2. NEO-HIPPIE
3. STREETER
4. DAÏKANYAMA LOLITA
5. PORNO CHIC LOLITA
6. SHOPPER
7. ROCKER
8. PIN-UP
9. CLASSIC CHIC

Definition by Rebecca Leach

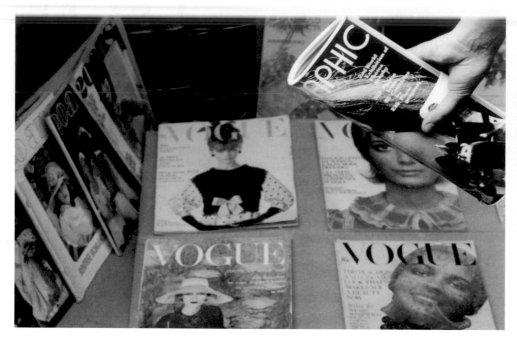

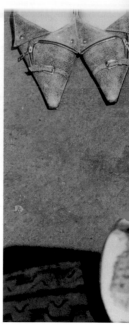

The fashion stylist works very closely with fashion magazines and photographers. A stylist is not a designer but an interpreter of fashion who puts together the concept of the looks for the photographs. He, or she, can also coordinate the fashion show looks, as well as working as a personal shopper (see Chapter 1, p. 31).

Magazines

The stylist organises the shots for editorials. The garments are displayed, ironed and tried on the models in the studio. After discussions with the hairdresser and make-up artist, the stylist will use pins to adjust the garment onto the model so that it fits perfectly. A stylist must always have their little box of tools so that the garments can be invisibly altered.

Celebrities

Whether it is a question of dressing a musician for a CD cover, or for coordinating an actor's wardrobe for special events (festivals, award ceremonies, etc.), the stylist must find the most suitable look for that person's personality and morphology. As these people are not mannequins, it is most important that the garment looks its best, but also that the person feels comfortable, and not self-conscious, when wearing it.

Promotion

The stylist will also organise shots for catalogues, press packs and advertising, making sure the client's brand is foremost.

There is an art in adapting to the client's taste – an attribute which the stylist must possess. For catalogue shoots, the stylist also arranges the settings and décor. The press pack shots, which present the entire collection to the press, are very similar to those of the catalogues.

In the case of advertising, the stylist works in the spirit of the costume designer: he or she creates the style corresponding to the staged character's identity.

Fashion show organisation

Here the stylist's job is to coordinate the looks, organise the casting of the models, choose the lighting, select the music etc., and sometimes help backstage with the dressers, make-up and hairdressers.

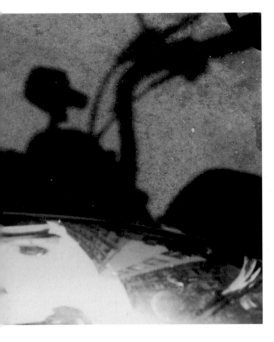
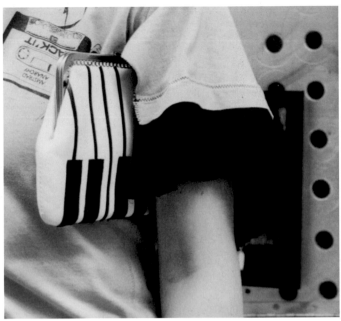

They can also be enlisted to send out invitations, buy accessories, underwear, small items such as tights, inner soles etc. and even manage part or all of the budget allocated to the models.

Consultation

Companies and designers will call on stylists for their ideas and knowledge about current fashion trends. At this point, they can inform the designer about the 'best of' products which could have been initially overlooked. The price, however, of a consultation can be quite high.

Rebecca Leach, alias Molly Coddle, has worked as a stylist in Paris for seven years. Graduating from the Metropolitan University of Manchester where she studied fashion history, she wrote a thesis on the alternative youth culture and their dress codes.

Fashion styling is a visual language, an art which helps one understand the human condition better. My sources of information stem from the internet sites of press offices, young designers and 'style.com'. As for buying, I choose according to my taste. I store the gathered information in a summary file on my computer, then contact the PR departments of the selected brands to see whether the clothes are available. Once the products are received, both clothes and accessories, I organise my looks.

This process of coordination does not follow any specific rules. Each fashion stylist has their own signature or trade mark - Camille Bidault-Waddington, Hector Castro (two stylists with very specific approaches), L'Wren Scott, or Carine Roitfeld, for example, all have individual and different styles.

For a fashion photo shoot, it is important to link all the elements illustrating the theme, so that the photographer has enough material to create his or her image. The cut, proportions, colour and texture of the proposed garments are chosen as a consequence thereof.

The opposite is also possible - the stylist can ask the photographer to react to a theme imposed by him or her. The key to a successful shot is good solid preparation.

Fashion photography

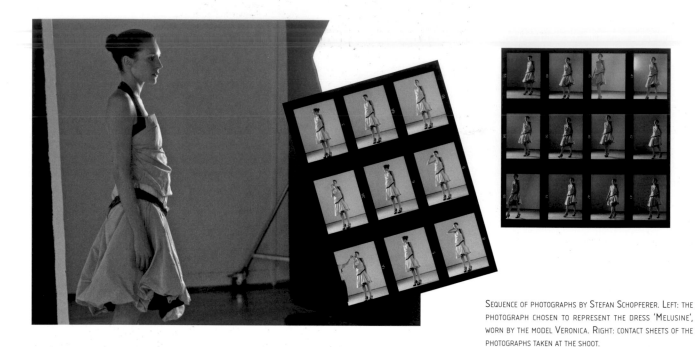

SEQUENCE OF PHOTOGRAPHS BY STEFAN SCHOPFERER. LEFT: THE PHOTOGRAPH CHOSEN TO REPRESENT THE DRESS 'MELUSINE', WORN BY THE MODEL VERONICA. RIGHT: CONTACT SHEETS OF THE PHOTOGRAPHS TAKEN AT THE SHOOT.

Specialities

The fashion photographer works for fashion magazines, advertising agencies, designer campaigns, etc. and is chosen for his, or her, style whether it be classic, commercial or avant-garde.

The basic journey of a photographer is in three stages: photography school, then assistant in a photo studio or with a photographer, where he/she applies all his/her knowledge putting it into reality and, finally, independent practice where his/her individual style can be honed and refined.

He/she can also fulfil the position of artistic director, like Olivier Toscani with Benetton, who favours the concept of marketing and whose shocking images and anti-racist messages are, strictly speaking, no longer fashion photographs.

A fashion photographer can be specialised in a variety of fields such as portrait, advertising, still life, art photography etc.

Celebrity photos of Bjork, Madonna, Nicole Kidman, or sporting personalities, such as David Beckham, resemble fashion shots more than they do simple portraits. However, Mario Testino is a fashion photographer who is perhaps better known for his pictures of Lady Di than for his fashion photographs.

There is a fine line between fashion and art photography. The numerous exhibitions devoted to fashion photographers by art galleries and museums bear witness to this with works of Jurgen Teller, Mario Sorrenti, and Steven Klein. However, the stolen snapshot, spontaneous and not touched-up are also in vogue.

Advertising photography stages models wearing designer labels, with the sole purpose of promoting the products for the consumer. The desired image is that of perfection, making sure the garment is shown off to its best advantage. On the other hand, fashion photography which has been inspired by still life has to portray garments, or products, without models. This type of informative photography tends to be used for catalogues and press packs.

In addition to this, fashion photographers can make a series of fashion compilations for magazines where the models are not staged but going about their everyday business.

The support team

For a shoot, the photographer, stylist, model, hair and make-up stylists and photo assistant must be able to work as a team.

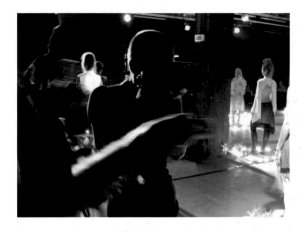

The approach varies depending on which type of magazine is targeted i.e. independent or conventional, with a fashion supplement (tie-up), catalogue or press pack.

Independent magazines, such as *Techni Art*, are creative and will allow the photography team to express themselves freely. The photographer aims to recreate an atmosphere, provoke a reaction and create an identity – in this instance, the clothes accessorise the photo. The same freedom of expression exists with certain press promotions such as those of Gucci, Yohji Yamamoto, Comme des Garçons and Dior, whose last advertising campaigns were carried out by Nick Knight. Photography must, first and foremost, inform the public about the brand. In this situation, the photographer and stylist work together to define the atmosphere and setting. The place for the shoot needs to be decided whether it be in a studio, inside (apartment, café, hotel room etc.) or outside (town, countryside, beach...). The photographer chooses the lighting (flash, daylight etc.) and the staging (dramatic, natural, experimental etc.). The choice of model is very important as it is he or she who brings the concept to life. The hair and make-up stylists' respective talents are put into practice and a brainstorming, with the whole team, takes place prior to the shoot.

For large distribution fashion magazines, catalogues and press packs, where the last collection, or a new season's trends are presented, the garment is central to the photo. The photographer and team work in conjunction with the client, who will have the final word concerning his product!

The shoot

The number of photos and days dedicated to the shoot varies depending on the client's demands, the support team and the preparations required for the photograph. It can vary from between 2 to 25 shots a day. Advertising photos, particularly beauty shots which require a lot of work with make-up, hair and lighting, take the most time. On the other hand, a series of 6 to 10- page fashion editorial will take one to two days. However, in the case of a special edition or particular magazine, the number of photos and days set aside for the shoot will vary accordingly.

For catalogues and press packs, the photographer will do 10 to 25 shots per day. There is less modification per shot, the studio lights are barely altered and it is rare to change venue for the outside shots; hair and make-up tends to stay the same.

As with a lot of jobs today, the work of a photographer has developed with the advent of new technologies. Digital photography has introduced a new approach with computer-enhanced images being increasingly more desired. The result is somehow not placed in reality. However, to

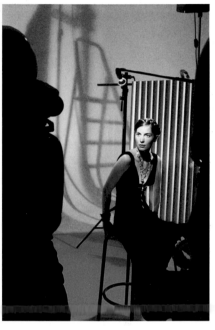

PHOTOGRAPHER JULES HERMANT TAKING A PHOTOGRAPH OF MODEL ALI MADHAVI AT A SHOOT FOR THE FOR THE LOULOU DE LA FALAISE AUTUMN/WINTER PRESS CATALOGUE. THE MODEL IS LUCIE DE LA FALAISE. HAIR BY KATIA AND VALENTINI. MAKE UP BY TANIA GANDRE. STYLIST ELIE TOP.

our eyes it has now become the norm. Skin appears softer and unwrinkled and bodies possess a dream-like perfection.

Photo sessions : make-up
Stéphane Marais, Beata Rosinska

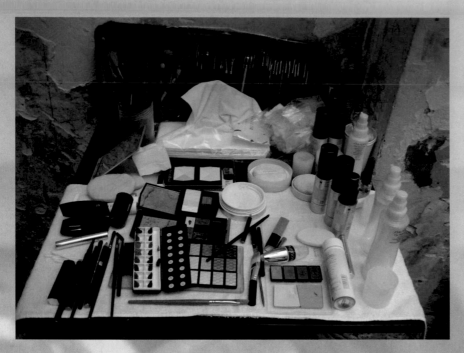

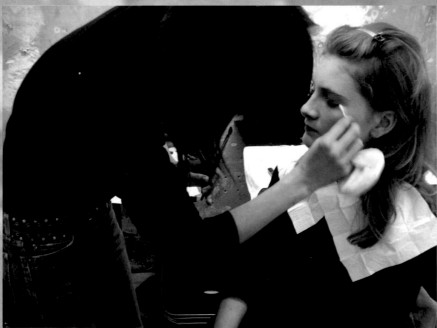

The art of make-up renders the models almost perfect for the catwalk or photo shoots. Certain make-up artists have such a distinct style that it becomes their signature. This being the case with Stéphane Marais who has worked with numerous photographers; Peter Lindbergh, Paolo Roversi, Irvin Penn, Annie Leibovitz, David Simms, Michael Thomson and Steven Klein, for international fashion magazines such as *Vogue*, *Harper's Bazaar*, *W Magazine*, and with the fashion stylist Frank Benhamou for the covers of the magazine *Numero*. He also worked with famous designers on the catwalk such as Lanvin, Lacroix, Gaultier, Comme des Garçons, Issey Miyake, Victor and Rolf, to name a few.

In an interview*, Stéphane Marais states that he is interested in working with all skin types – black, white and Asian: He is quoted as saying 'I am interested in ethnic groups which have long been ignored'. His make-up is the result of extensive research, for example, his interest in the Nouba tribes of the Sudan has inspired some of his fashion show work. It is essential to have a good grasp of general culture in order to understand the stylist and reinforce the themes which are being presented.

Stéphane Marais prefers natural looking make-up which allows the model's skin to show through. According to him a successful makeup is one 'which gives the illusion of being invisible, as if one has taken most of it off just after it has been applied'.

He makes a Polaroid record of each of his catwalk make-up sessions, a choice of which can be found in his publication *Beauty Flash* (Editions 7L – 2001).

* France Japan éco, *été 2002*

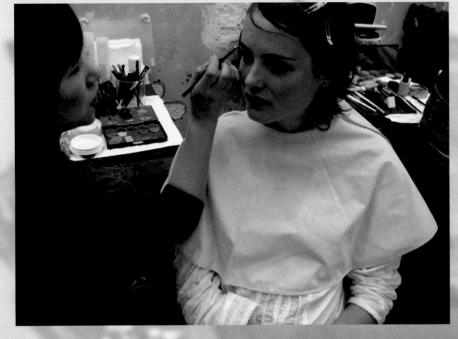

For make-up and hair stylist, Beata Rosinska, ex-assistant to Nina Haverkamp (Jed Root agency) and to Ashley Ward (Watson Agency) in London, the skin is also the most important part of make-up. She chooses invisible, delicate, luminous foundations and avoids applying them around the eye area. Then she concentrates on the parts of the face which are the most inspiring: the mouth, the eyes, the cheekbones.... ' I prefer delicate and transparent textures which do not look over-loaded.'

The second stage is to correct the under-eye shadows with a cream that is fixed by a light dusting of powder. This lightens and rejuvenates the face.

Blusher is the final stage, which gives structure and definition to the face, as well as correcting any blemishes and giving it a radiant complexion. The most important factor being that the make up looks harmonious.

Naturally, she changes her style to suit the different designers and clothing without losing sight of the spirit, or theme, of the show. For cinema photography, the 'rules' are stricter, particularly taking into account the lighting.

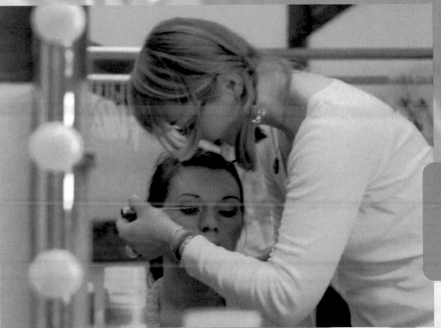

BACKSTAGE AT THE PRESENTATION OF THE SPRING/SUMMER '07 COLLECTION BY LUTZ.
LEFT AND ABOVE: MAKE-UP SESSION OF VERONICA BY BEATA ROSINSKA.

Interview with Odile Gilbert

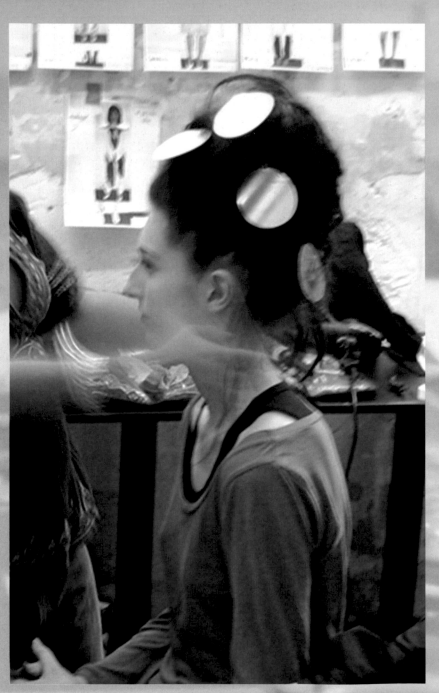

Hair styling has become a complete art with Odile Gilbert, who, for more than 20 years has demonstrated her talent and skill in the world media. Supreme recognition came when on the 12th July 2006, she was made a Knight of the Order of Les Arts et des Lettres of the French Republic. She belongs to that generation of top models such as Naomi Campbell, Linda Evangelista, Claudia Schieffer etc....

Her rich experience with Chanel, Lacroix, Gaultier, Hermès, Rochas, Celine, Botegga, Veneta etc. has meant that she is constantly reviewing her inventive approach to hair dressing whether it be for a fashion show or a photo session. 'Hair is alive, that is its beauty' she told us.

Odile Gilbert began her career as an assistant in 1975 in Bruno Pittini's hair salon and studio. 'Hair stylists must study the techniques and chemical compositions necessary for colours and perms in a hair dressing school. Mastering the various cutting techniques, perms, straightening and hair extensions is the result of a rigorous apprenticeship and very necessary in order to adapt to the individual identity of each fashion house.' This rigour has been proved by her work with houses as diverse as Chanel, Gaultier and Lacroix.

In preparation for the fashion show, the first step is to have a discussion with the stylist. This is a question of 'translat-

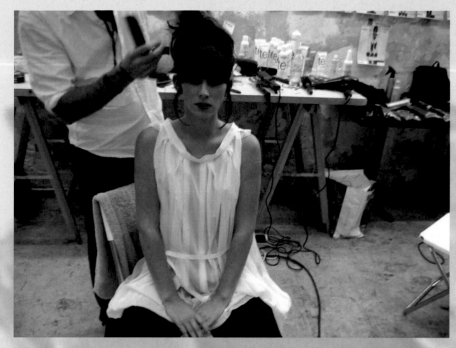

BACKSTAGE AT THE PRESENTATION OF THE SPRING/SUMMER COLLECTION 2007 BY LUTZ.

ing the theme of the collection' into the hairstyles and help to 'find a balance between the silhouette and the proportions'. This analysis is critical to fashion culture because to design a silhouette is, in fact, to create a woman. Odile describes hair styling 'as a form of architecture where one strikes a balance between the overall effect of lines, material and volume'.

The fashion shows have allowed her to express her creativity widely. However, she is quick to extend her appreciation of the collaborative aspect of this work, in particular, when working on numerous advertising campaigns (for Lagerfield Gallery, Sonia Rykiel, Yohji Yamamoto etc.). For her, the photographs are 'the result of team work between the stylist, make-up artist, hair stylist, photographer and model who combine their talents with the aim of creating an image'.

Odile Gilbert has published a compilation of her creations *Her Style*, which has been prefaced by Karl Lagerfeld (Éditions 7L, 2003).

HAIRSTYLING FOR VÉRONICA BY BEATA ROSINSKA.

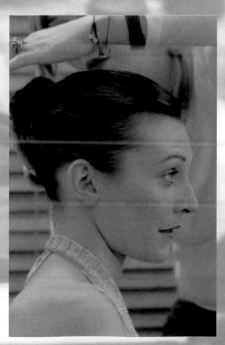

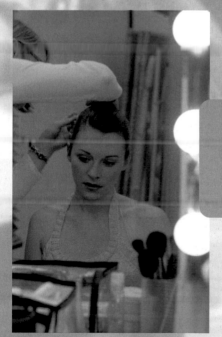

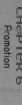

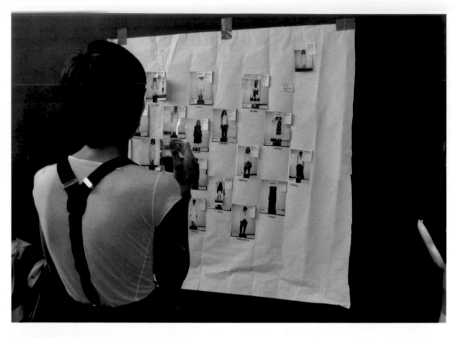

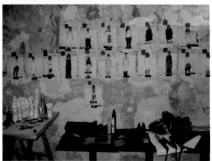

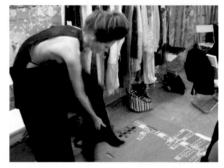

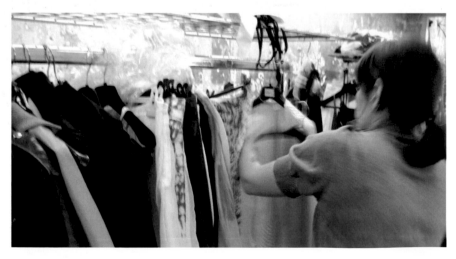

The fashion show is the event where a brand's next season collection is presented to the professionals, press, photographers, buyers and VIP clients.

Large brands such as Chanel can finance large *prêt-à-porter* shows with up to 220 garments.

A show can range from being extremely spectacular, like those of John Galliano for Dior, to a simple presentation. Lutz prefers short shows of 25 looks coordinating strong pieces (which make a statement about the brand image) with simple elements, such as jumpers or accessories, chosen from some 60 items, of which 30 are woven and 30 are knitwear. He prefers not to have just 'show pieces' which have been exclusively reserved for the fashion show.

Everything that Lutz presents exists in the shops. He states: 'For a small concern the aim is to make garments which really sell, as well as make an impression on the catwalk.'

For a long time, he used modelling agencies to supply his fashion shows but now he prefers to recruit amateur models who he comes across at parties or events and whose style corresponds to the collection in question.

For Lutz, the choice of make-up artist is central to the concept of his collection. 'Make-up is a form of communication. It confirms the style of the woman

HERE AND ON THE FOLLOWING PAGES: FINAL PREPARATIONS FOR LUTZ'S SPRING-SUMMER COLLECTION 2007. THE MODELS' LOOKS ARE CHECKED, DÉCOR PUT IN PLACE AND THE SOUND-TRACK TESTED.

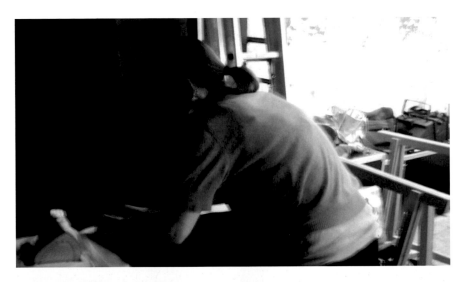

chosen for the collection. It accentuates a certain model's traits or, conversely, can make the model "disappear" in order to place more emphasis on the clothes. This is the same with hair styling.'

The choice of music is decided once the collection has been finished. It is the final touch. In Lutz's case, he chooses the music and his sound engineer, Michel Gaubert, mixes the sound-track. He remembers having intentionally selected the entire 12 inch album of Donna Summer's *Love to love you baby* for one of his fashion shows. 'Certain designers prefer very rhythmic music for their shows, others obscure it in their desire to surprise. However, music must not automatically respond to the public's expectations. The designer must also be able to express himself outside of the garment.'

Backstage, in the wings of the fashion show, the clothes to be worn by the models on the catwalk are hung up on a rail. A sequence board displays the different turns which are numbered and identified by Polaroid shots.

Each model has his or her own dresser. These last finishing details are carried out amongst a jostling bustle of make-up artists, hair stylists, designers, models and photographers whilst journalists penetrate this mythical place and attempt to snatch interviews and photos.

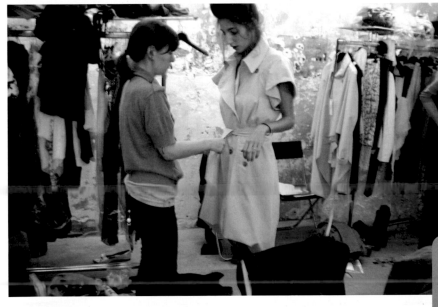

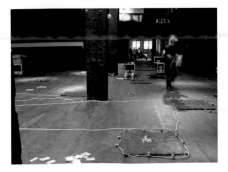

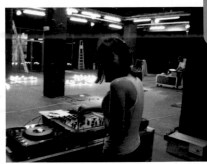

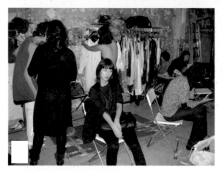
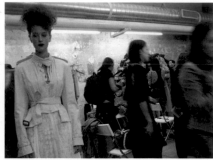
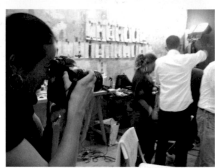
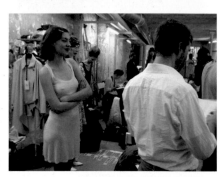
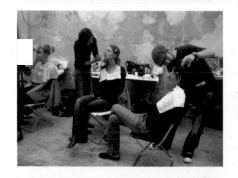
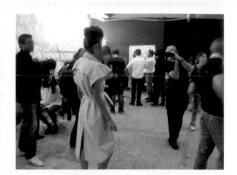
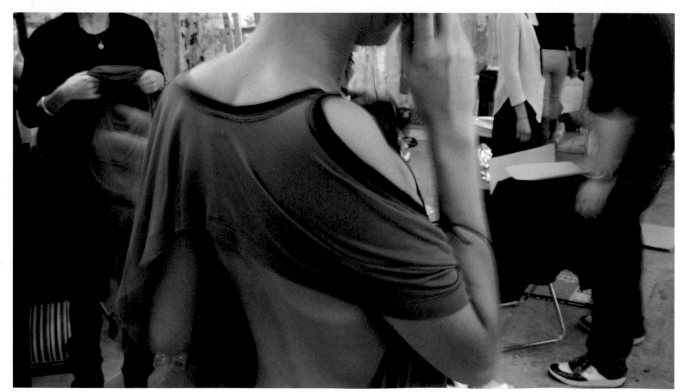

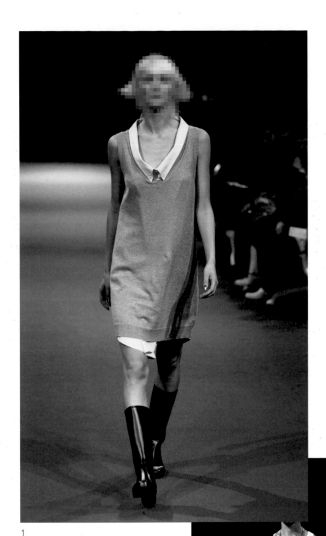

1

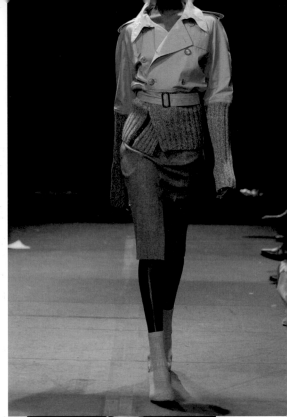

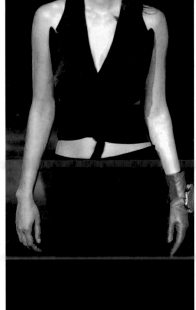

2

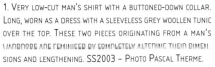

4

1. VERY LOW-CUT MAN'S SHIRT WITH A BUTTONED-DOWN COLLAR. LONG, WORN AS A DRESS WITH A SLEEVELESS GREY WOOLLEN TUNIC OVER THE TOP. THESE TWO PIECES ORIGINATING FROM A MAN'S WARDROBE ARE FEMINISED BY COMPLETELY ALTERING THEIR DIMENSIONS AND LENGTHENING. SS2003 – PHOTO PASCAL THERME.

2. CUT-OUT FLOWER IN SILK BROCADE TOP, WORN OVER A MAN'S SLEEVELESS COTTON TANK TOP AND GREY SKIRT WITH EMBROIDERED SEQUINS. GARDENING ANKLE BOOTS IN SHINY BLACK PLASTIC. SS 2003 – PHOTO PASCAL THERME.

3. MINI-TRENCH COAT WITH KNITWEAR EXTENSIONS. A 'CUT AND PASTE' ITEM CREATING A SPECIFIC MIX, VERY MUCH IN THE STYLE OF LUTZ. AW 2004-2005- PHOTO PASCAL THERME.

4. NEW LOOK SMOKING WAISTCOAT. AW 2007 – PHOTO PASCAL THERME.

appendices

DRAWING AND SEWING EQUIPMENT

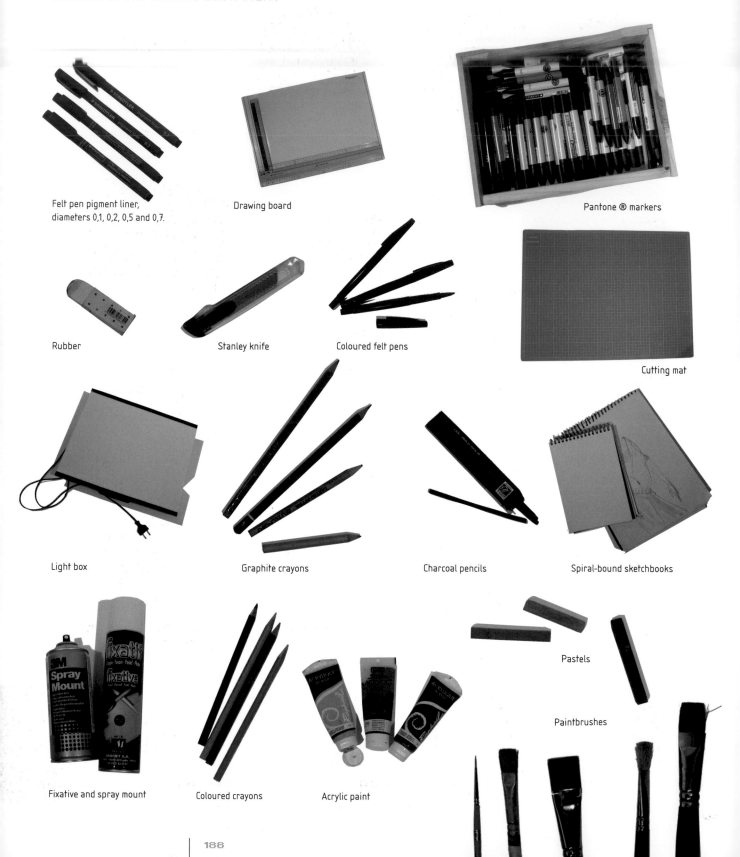

Felt pen pigment liner,
diameters 0,1, 0,2, 0,5 and 0,7.

Drawing board

Pantone ® markers

Rubber

Stanley knife

Coloured felt pens

Cutting mat

Light box

Graphite crayons

Charcoal pencils

Spiral-bound sketchbooks

Fixative and spray mount

Coloured crayons

Acrylic paint

Pastels

Paintbrushes

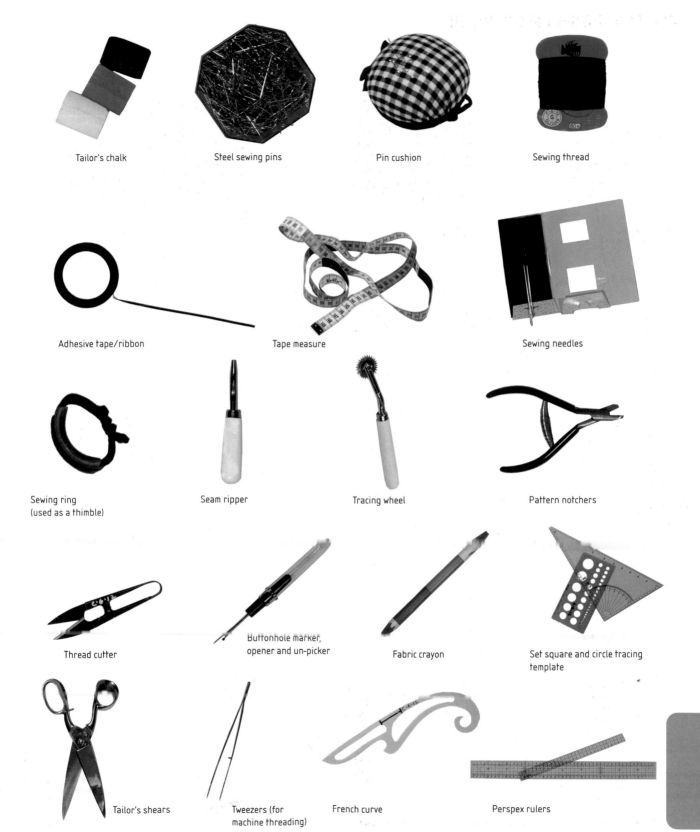

Tailor's chalk

Steel sewing pins

Pin cushion

Sewing thread

Adhesive tape/ribbon

Tape measure

Sewing needles

Sewing ring
(used as a thimble)

Seam ripper

Tracing wheel

Pattern notchers

Thread cutter

Buttonhole marker,
opener and un-picker

Fabric crayon

Set square and circle tracing
template

Tailor's shears

Tweezers (for
machine threading)

French curve

Perspex rulers

appendices

MINI DICTIONARY OF MATERIALS AND MACHINES

MATERIALS

ACETATE

Synthetic fibres obtained from pure cellulose (cotton or wood pulp). Its name is derived from one of its components, acetic acid, and it can be known as cellulose acetate. Acetate threads can be used in viscose, cotton or silk weaves. As well as being found in delicate fabrics it is also found in denser fabrics such as taffetas, twills and satin. One of the principal qualities being its 'fall', which lends itself to being used in net and curtain production, as well as simulating silk and linings.

ACRYLIC

Acrylic fibres are amongst some of the lightest synthetic fibres. They can be used pure or mixed with other fabrics such as cotton or wool. They allow for the manufacture of quick drying, non-creasing garments which do not require ironing: it is for these reasons that they are found in sportswear, streetwear and work clothing.

BATIK

Printed cotton fabric originating from the islands of Java and Sumatra and the East Indies, where the word *batikken* means 'drawn by hand'. After having drawn onto a fabric, wax is applied to certain areas to prevent them from being dyed, as a form of resist-dyeing. This material is characterised by bright colours and geometric patterns.

BATISTE

Originally a sheer, finely woven cloth of brushed cotton or linen. It is now the generic name for a sheer, fine, mercerised cotton used for baby clothes, blouses, dresses and lingerie.

BAZIN

Usually one colour cotton printed fabric originating from Africa (see Wax Fabrics).

BENGALINE

Viscose material, with small ribs, obtained by weaving cloth with the weft threads slightly slackened. The ribs are more pronounced than poplins and more regular than Ottoman fabrics. It is a dense and reversible material, used for furnishing fabrics and clothing (jackets, dresses and skirts).

BIRDSEYE

A worsted suiting type of fabric, featuring a small design based on a diamond with a small dot in the centre of the pattern (similar to a 'bird's eye'). It is achieved by a combination of weave and colour. Used mainly for suits.

BROCADE

From the Italian *broccato*. Originating from luxurious silk fabrics decorated with stitched patterns using gold or silver threads which give the impression of a raised design. It is woven and produced with a supplementary, non-structural weft thread in addition to the standard weft threads that hold the warp together. Nowadays, these patterns are made using the jacquard method with silk and /or metallic threads. Brocade is associated with evening wear and furnishing fabrics.

CALICO

Natural plain weave cotton cloth deriving its name from the village of Calicut in India. It is un-dyed and rough in texture; being used for bed linen (under sheets, etc.) as well as for the *toiles* of garment prototypes. It is also used as the background cloth of traditionally printed fabrics of native Americans and Indians. In this instance, calico is called Indian *toile*.

CASHMERE

The combings of the undercoat hair of mountain goats from Mongolia and the Himalayas. The wool is very precious and used for creating very fine, warm and luxurious fabric for coats and knitwear. It is also a fibre of Indian origin, which can be used pure or mixed to produce shawls with characteristic designs; the term cashmere can also mean a type of pattern or motif.

CELLULOSE

Cellulose is the principal constituent of every vegetable fibre and is the most widespread of all the natural organic materials. Being of capital importance for traditional as well as industrial textiles, the fibres are found in cotton, linen, jute and hemp. After undergoing chemical treatment, cellulose produces acetate, viscose and other synthetic fibres.

CHAMBRAY (see Pinpoint Oxford)

A type of yarn-dyed, plain weave cotton fabric with a coloured, or indigo, warp and a white, or beige, weft: the overall effect is that of denim-like effect. Its lightweight makes it easy to sew and gives a more interesting fall to the fabric. Due to this, jean shirts and children's clothes are made from this.

CHENILLE

This trimming, or fabric, derives its name from the French word meaning caterpillar as its soft, fuzzy-looking yarns stand out around a velvet cord. It is obtained by cutting the velvet into very thin strips. It is often used as the thread for knitted cardigans and furnishing fabrics.

CHEVIOT

Originating from the sheep on the Cheviot hills in Scotland, this material is a type of carded wool with a rough, dense texture traditionally used for menswear.

CHEVRON

Generic term given to fabrics which form a 'V' pattern when assembled (similar to an alternate crossed twill weave). Chevron materials are normally used for coats, jackets and suits.

CHIFFON (see Crêpe)

CHINTZ

Derived from the Hindi word *chint* meaning 'printed fabric', today it refers to plain or floral printed woven cotton or viscose (or sometimes both) with a glazed or shiny side. Due to the fabric fall, it is normally used in furnishing fabrics but sometimes for summer dresses and skirts.

CLOQUE

A double fabric used in the manufacture of womenswear, with a 'blistered' effect produced by the use of yarns of a different character or twist making ridges on the inside of the material and which respond in different ways to finishing treatments.

COTTON

One of the most classic fibres obtained by weaving the downy fibre surrounding the seeds of the cotton plant. It is the most abundant and widespread fibre in the world; it is tough, silky and easy to work and dye. Delicate and light, or heavy and dense, cotton products are used in a variety of fabrics and garments either on their own or mixed with other natural or synthetic fibres:

American Cotton: variety of ordinary cotton produced in the United States.
Egyptian Cotton: produced in Egypt, the Sudan and Mali; this cotton has a longer fibre and is of a better quality.
Cotton and Silk: (see Silk and Cotton (Silk))
Honeycomb cotton: (see Crêpe (Crépon))
Cotton Cloth: printed cotton plain weave cloth used in the manufacture of summer clothes, aprons and furnishing fabrics.

CRASH

Plain weave fabric originally obtained from flax. Today it is made from linen, cotton or rayon and used in the manufacture of suits.

CRÈPE

Originating from the Latin word crispus meaning 'frizzy' and subsequently, the French word crêper meaning to 'crimp' or 'frizz', this term is used to describe all fabrics which have a crinkly, crimped or grained texture. This is obtained by a particular weave effect or by using threads under a strong tension. The fabric can also acquire this crimped texture, after weaving, by chemical or thermal treatment.
Chiffon: very light, delicate woven fabric, mixed with silk threads and synthetic fibres, used for evening dresses, blouses and scarves.
Crêpe De Chine: Medium weight silk, or polyester, of which the warp is made from raw threads (beige or natural coloured originating from the silk cocoon) and the weft from crêpe threads. When it is light and dense, it is called lingerie crêpe; if the weft is made with thick crêpe thread then it is termed Moroccan crêpe.

Georgette Crèpe: a sheer, lightweight plain weave fabric with a fine crepe texture. Softer and more transparent than Crepe de Chine. It is composed of very tightly tensioned threads. Its lightness and delicacy lends itself ideally to evening dresses and camisoles.

Woollen Crèpe: its woollen weft makes the fabric soft and delicate, however, it is very strong to the touch. It can be used for suits and dresses.

Satin-Backed Crèpe: satin weave fabric. The right side is lustrous whereas the reverse is matt. Its lightness and fall makes it ideal for dresses, blouses and lingerie.

Crèpon (Or Honeycomb Cotton): it can be 100% cotton or mixed with other fabrics. Its principal characteristics being its crinkled or puckered nature, with a more prominent fluted effect in the warp direction giving a tree bark effect. Its lightness means it is used for summer dresses and camisoles.

CROCHET

Loose, open knitwear made using a small, curved knitting needle, resembling a musical crochet. Giving wool a light, characteristic quality, it can be used for summer sweaters, as well as baby clothes. This term can equally be used for clothes made from copper, steel or even wood, using in this method. Crochet effects can now be made by machines.

CROSSED (or DENSE TEXTURE)

Cotton fabric and/or mixed fibres where the twill weave gives a slanted effect on the right-side of the fabric, as well as on the reverse.

DAMASK

Self-coloured complex weave fabric (either satin, twill or plain weave) which owes its name to Damascus in Syria. It is generally a satin, figured pattern on a taffeta, woollen or silk background. Its main characteristic being its reversibility so that, on one side, the patterns are matt with the background being lustrous and, on the other side, the reverse. It is used in clothing, furnishing and bed covers. In addition to this, the term 'damasked' can mean all fabrics which have reversible patterns which are alternately matt and shiny.

DENIM

Cotton fabric which owes its name to the city of Nimes in France where it is thought to have originated. It is characterised by its twill weave with indigo warp threads and white or, natural, weft ones. Its flexibility and hardwearing meant that is became the archetypal American work clothing in the 1930s and nowadays is synonymous with jean material the world over.

DEVORÉ

Derived from the French word devoré to mean eaten, it is applied to luxury fabrics where some of the surface has been, either acid-etched, or burnt away to create the decoration.

DOBBY

Fabric produced on a loom sharing the same name, i.e. a dobby attachment, with narrow strips of wood instead of Jacquard cards. Dobby weaves are complex (satin, twill or plain weaves) with simple, small, repeatable all-over designs and are used for blouses and shirts.

DOUBLE FACE

This is a generic term for any reversible fabric made from different coloured and contrasting warps and wefts.

DUCK CLOTH

Cotton fabric with a half hopsack weave. Its thickness and strength means it is suitable for sportswear, work clothing and accessories (shoes, bags etc.).

EMBROIDERY

Strands of coloured silk or woollen threads sewn onto a fabric to produce a given motif. Embroidery was originally done by hand, using sewing needles, and is still the case with haute couture items when pearls and sequins are added. For industrially produced garments, there has been a significant growth in computer-assisted embroidery.

FAILLE

Coming from the Flemish word *falie*, this is a dressy, ribbed fabric with a light lustre originally made in taffetas (silk) with rounded and horizontal ribs, the effect being due to the alternate weft threads being of variable widths. Today, faille is normally synthetic made from an acetate, polyester or viscose base. Its lustre and delicacy means it is suitable for women's dresses, suits etc.

FALSE FUR

Made from an acrylic base, this fabric can be knitted or woven, dyed one colour or printed. Used for the manufacture of coats, linings or trimmings

FANCY YARNS

Grenadine: very fine silk thread, principally used for hand-made, *haute couture* items. It is reputed to be the finest thread in the world.

Lamé: originally thread made from metal (gold, silver or copper). Nowadays it is made from filaments of coloured polyester film.

FELT

Obtained from strands of wool, or other animal hair, belonging to the section of non-woven, non-spun materials. The technique of felting is still traditionally practised by nomadic populations in the Far East. In the textile industry, felting is done mechanically using heat and humidity to produce the material.

FIGURED

This term describes the generic way every complex-weave fabric with small Jacquard patterns is done. It is used for blouses and dresses.

FIL-A-FIL/YARN ON YARN

A woven fabric where a white thread is interwoven with a coloured one end to end and characterised by a diagonal step pattern. This process is often used for poplin.

FLANNEL

A durable woollen (but sometimes cotton) woven fabric. There are several types (tennis flannels, partially or completely dyed.) Its strong yet soft texture lends it to skirt and trouser manufacture as well as suits, jackets, their collars and linings.

FLOCKING

Downy pattern or motif in relief, made by the 'flocking' technique. This consists of laying down an adhesive onto the basic fabric and applying small textile fibres onto the sticky area. Used in the making of blouses, dresses and furnishing fabrics and street or sportswear logos etc.

FRENCH TERRY CLOTH

Cotton fabric made from a double warp thread: the first one is taught and the second is slack. After beating, one will become the background and the other the loop. Decorative patterns can be obtained by inserting coloured threads (machinery-made Jacquard) before beating the two warps.

GABARDINE

From the Spanish word *gabardina* and the old French *gavardine*, meaning coat. Durable, tightly woven cotton or wool fabric made in a twill weave with distinct diagonal ribs. Its woollen texture renders it naturally waterproof making it a suitable fabric for raincoats, sportswear, suits and uniforms.

GAUZE

Thin, translucent fabric with loose open weave, originally cotton, coming from the town of Gaza in Palestine. Today this material is made from wool or silk and with its light, delicate qualities is used in the production of blouses and dresses.

GINGHAM CHECK

Fresh, light plain weave cotton fabric. Due to the way it is woven, this fabric's main characteristic is the alternating white and coloured threads giving squares of varying sizes. It is used in the manufacture of children's clothes, shirts, blouses, as well as bed linen and furnishings.

GUIPURE

Machine-embroidered lace which characterised by appearing to be without a background.
The patterns are separated by spaces which have either been dissolved or cut out from the base material.

HORSEHAIR

Dense canvas made with a cotton warp thread and a horsehair weft thread. Used in menswear clothing.

HOUND'S (DOG) TOOTH CLOTH

Twill weave with lozenge-shaped checks made by alternating the colours of the warp and weft. Available in varying sizes of check. Normally used for the manufacture of suits, coats and accessories such as bags, scarves etc.).

INTEGRATED PRINTED PATTERN

Fabric on which a pattern/motif can be printed repetitively, covering the entire fabric (all over pattern), positioned just on the border (integrated printed pattern) or just on a specific area of the garment (placed motif).

INTERLOCK

The characteristic of this fabric is that it knit stitches interconnect with the weft making a thicker and heavier ply. It has a more natural stretch than a jersey knit and the same appearance and feel on both sides. It is fine, easy to cut and sew. It is used for dresses, tee-shirts and leggings as well as for underwear.

JACQUARD

The name is derived from the inventor of this mechanical weaving method, Joseph M. Jacquard. The fabric is one, or multi-, coloured presenting bands of geometric patterns which can vary infinitely. The pattern is punched into a pasteboard, each row corresponding to one row of the design, which guides the warp thread so that the weft thread will lie above or below it. Most often, a jumper with crossed, coloured threads is a jersey. Used for suits, jackets or skirts.

JERSEY

This knitwear fabric, originally made from wool, was used to make sailor's jumpers in the island of Jersey, Channel Islands. Today it is a generic term used to describe any fabric made by simple weaving, without any obvious ribs. Used for sportswear, dresses and tee-shirts.

Matt Jersey: Matte and dull knit fabric made with very fine crepe yarns. Used for slinky eveningwear.

Velvet Jersey: weft knit having a velvet aspect on the right side and flat on the reverse.

KNITTING

This generic term encompasses every fabric which is made from linked loops of yarn. It is divided into two large groups, weft knitting and warp knitting (hybrid of knitting and weaving using a beam of warp threads linked together by a moving rack of needles).

2 X 2 Rib Knitting: ribbed weft knit, very stretchy. Used for pullovers and cardigans.

Polar Or Brushed Knit: double weft knit, one colour or printed, brushed on both faces with a quilted texture. Most often made from polyester, it is used for pullovers, sportswear, accessories and linings.

Single Jersey Knit: warp knit with a light lustrous texture used for lingerie and blouses.

Double Jersey Knit: double weft knit, also known as 'interlock' dense as though woven, used for dresses, suits, jackets and trousers.

Terry Towelling Knit: weft knit looped on the right side, used for baby clothes, beachwear and sportswear.

Jacquard Knit: Double jersey patterned knit using as many as four colours in a row; usually programmed and controlled by computerised machinery.

Cavalry Twill or Tricotine: weft knit in twill weave, often wool, used for uniforms, coats and trousers.

LINEN

The linen fibre comes from the flax plant. Linen cloth is one of the oldest textiles in the world and has been known for centuries in Asia and Egypt where it is considered a 'noble' material. Modern techniques of treating the stalks, such as 'scutching' (removing the woody portions of the stalk by crushing them between two metal rollers) and 'hackling' (combing the short fibres away to leave the long, soft flax fibres), allows the fabric to range from soft and supple to stiff and rough. Used for shirts, skirts and jackets.

LINON

This fabric derives its name from linen, as it was originally woven using the flax plant fibres. Plain weave, slightly broken, this fabric is so fine it is semi-transparent.

Today, it exists in cotton and ramie. It is mostly printed and used for bodices, flat collars, cuffs, summer dresses and babies underwear.

White Linon: also called opal. This is fine, slightly transparent and very soft. It is used for blouses and night clothes (pyjamas, nightshirts etc.).

LODEN

This is a thick, water-resistant fabric made from sheep's wool which has been boiled and carded then plain woven. It is well-known in Bavaria where it is used as coat and suit material.

LUSTRE

Plain weave fabric, generally in brushed wool or mohair, which is light yet strong; used for summer suits.

LYCRA

In 1959 Dupont de Nemours's registered this trademark for its brand of elastomer. It is a very light fabric with great elasticity used for running and sportswear.

MADRAS

This cotton weft fabric with its simple texture owes its name to the town in India from which it originates. Large squares or multi-coloured designs are very characteristic of this plain weave fabric. The bright colours and lightness of this fabric lends itself to traditional headdresses worn in the Antilles.

MARQUISETTE

A sheer gauze fabric which is light and transparent and sometimes made from silk, cotton or synthetic fibres. Used for lingerie and dresses and furnishing fabrics, in particular, for mosquito nets, net curtains etc.

MATELASSÉ

A double cloth with a quilted appearance commonly made with two warps and two wefts. The quilted effect can be accentuated by the use of wadding threads and the designs are formed by floating threads or small areas of waves. It is also a generic term used for the linings of coats and jackets and can be used as stuffing, or wadding, as in 'Puffa' jackets etc.

MELTON

A thick to medium thick tightly woven wool with a heavily brushed nap giving the fabric a smooth finish with no warp or weft visible similar to felt. Used in coat manufacture.

MICROFIBRE

Generic term used to describe all synthetic fibres – often from a polyester base – but finer than silk. Microfibre fabrics are soft, light, breathable and strong which means they can be suitable for all sorts of garments.

MILLERAIES

Brushed woollen fabric with many fine stripes used for suit manufacture.

MOIRÉ

This fabric originates from goat's hair. It is characterised by the wave reflections due to its weaving which, in places, crushes the fabric after having been folded in two. Generally, any fabric which has this undulating effect and it is used in the manufacture of blouses, dresses and evening wear.

MOLESKIN

A heavy quality brushed cotton used for trousers, jackets, dungarees and children's clothing. By brushing the reverse side of cotton cloth, a downy and warm quality is obtained. Moleskin is sometimes used as a coating on one side of a leather garment or shoe and so it can also refer to coated cloth.

MUSLIN

This fabric was originally made from silk (chiffon) or wool but nowadays is made from all sorts of materials such as wool, cotton (muslin) or rayon threads. It is extremely light, soft and semi-transparent. Woollen muslin is used for dresses with floral patterns whereas silk muslin, made with tight tension threads, is used for evening dresses, lingerie and camisoles.

NAPPED

This describes fabrics which can only be cut in one direction. Particularly important for printed fabrics such as madras or those with a definite 'hair' or pile, such as velvet.

NYLON

In 1935, Dupont de Nemours registered the trademark for this material and now its name, and the synthetic fibre (polyamide) from which it comes, is known throughout the world.

Today, nylon can be vinyl and cotton, or rayon. Its supreme elasticity lends itself to the manufacture of tights and stockings. It is also very absorbent.

OPENWORK

Woven or knitted fabric with an open structure, having a gauze or complex weave, i.e. where the warp and weft threads are spaced out.

ORGANDIE

Similar to muslin in that it is very light, delicate and transparent yet it is stiffer. It is a plain weave cotton which can be used for blouses, dresses, trimmings and net curtains.

ORGANZA

Plain weave fabric resembling organdie but made from silk or synthetic threads. Its uses are similar to those above.

OTTOMAN

This Turkish fabric is made using a woollen, silk or viscose warp. It is characterised by deep transversal ribs obtained by inserting supplementary wefts. Nowadays it refers to all fabrics which present this type of ribbing, whatever their finesse and regularities are (see Bengaline). They are normally used for coats and blazers.

PAGNE (see Wax)

Name given to the fabric made from vegetable fibres (raffia) which can also be made from cotton. The pattern is drawn onto the fabric and then painstakingly small holes are punched along the design lines. Hot wax then seals the image which has been dyed or painted. It is traditionally worn tied around the waist, up under the arms or tied at the nape of the neck in countries such as Africa, Asia, Caribbean. Its lightness and bright colours, once dyed, makes it suitable for the spring-summer collections of dresses, skirts, shirts, Bermudas and trousers.

PEAU-DE-PÊCHE

From the French word meaning 'peach skin', this fabric is similar to moleskin but is lighter and softer as it is made from micro-fibre weaves. Its downy texture is obtained by chemical treatment. It is normally used to make sweat tops for street and sportswear.

PIN STRIPE

Very fine 'pin-head' striped fabric.

PINPOINT OXFORD (see Chambray)

Lightweight, soft, cotton-like fabric with small 2x1 basket weave repeats. The warp threads are dyed whilst the wefts are left white – this creates a small ribbed pattern. Oxfords can be either striped or checked. As it is very easy to sew, its texture and fall make it very suitable for shirts and children's clothing.

PIQUÉ

A knitted cotton fabric with a waffle, or diamond shaped, pattern. Its weave is composed of two warps, one for the background the other for the stitches. French piqué knits became an international fashion when René Lacoste, the 1920s tennis champion, designed the short-sleeved polo shirt made from 100% cotton.

Bedford Piqué: This is made with vertical ribs on the right-side of the fabric. Used in children's clothing ands women's outdoor wear.

PLUMETIS

This is a fabric whose patterns are obtained by inserting extra warp or weft threads. It can also refer to a cloth with small relief patterns or motifs which could be embroidered, flocked or woven.

POINTELLE

Very delicate, feminine rib knit fabric made with relief eyelet patterns. Used for womenswear.

POPLIN

A durable, plain weave fabric made originally form a mix of natural silk warps and cotton or wool wefts. Today, poplin has fine horizontal lines due to the fact that the number of warp threads is double the number of weft threads. It is similar to broadcloth yet with a heavier rib and weight. Used primarily in high-quality shirt manufacture.

PRINCE OF WALES CHECK

Derived from the prince who popularised this material, Edward VII when he was Prince of Wales. Very large check with a repeat of nine inches in bold red or brown on a cream background with a grey over-check. Sometimes confused with the Edward, the Duke of Windsor's preference for Glen Urquhart's black and white check.

RABANNE

Material from Madagascar made from only the raffia fibres or occasionally mixed with synthetic fibres. Used in accessory manufacture such as hats and bags or furnishings.

RAFFIA

This Madagascan word refers to the vegetable fibre derived from the leaves of the palm trees found in Africa and the Indian Ocean. Being light makes it easy to weave and is used in the manufacture of place mats, table coverings and mats as well as decorative additions, with cotton, on dresses, shirts and accessories (bags, hats etc.).

RAYON (see artificial silk)

RIP-STOCK

A fabric woven with a double thread at regular intervals so that small tears do not become larger. Very useful in the manufacture of parachutes and tents, as well as sportswear.

SATEEN

This is the reverse of satin with a smooth weft face and is normally made from cotton. Used for blouses and dresses.

SATIN

The term is derived from the Chinese town of Zaytoun. It was originally a silk cloth where the warp dominated the weft. The weft is almost completely covered, giving a smooth face free from any twill with the main characteristic being a lustrous and glossy sheen. There are a great variety of satins: Chinese satin (shiny and smooth); Lyon satin (made in twill); Duchess satin (thick, heavy and very expensive) etc. Satins are most often made from silk, viscose or acetate and used for evening wear and costumes.

SCHIFFLI (embroidery)

This type of embroidery owes its name to the commercial embroidery machine, which uses a combination of a needle and shuttle to form a stitch. Vine-like floral patterns on sheer fabrics characterise this material. It is first embroidered by the machine, then the background material is 'melted' away using a chemical treatment. It is used for emblem production, lace creation and satin fabric embroidery.

SEERSUCKER

A term originating from the USA, it is characterised by the presence of flat and puckered sections, particularly in stripes and checks. The effect is produced in various ways, either by stripes with different tensions that cause crinkling, by using yarns with different shrinkages or by treating certain areas of the fabric causing it to shrink.

SHANTUNG

This fabric takes its name from the province in China from where it was originally made. It was hand-loomed and is thin and soft, woven with uneven yarns to produce an irregular surface. Twentieth-century shantung is usually made of silk mixed with cotton or rayon thus creating a heavier fabric than its original counterpart. Both fabrics are used for evening wear.

SHETLAND

Generic term referring to woollen fabrics originating from the sheep on the Scottish islands of Shetland. These materials are often woven or knitted and used for suits and coats.

SILK

Natural fibre produced the silkworm, a grub of the silk moth, which feeds on the mulberry tree. The worms spin cocoons exuding fine filaments forming a thread. Its production methods were kept secret for centuries. It originated in China and was bought to Europe around the 12th century along the 'silk routes' with the merchant traders. It has always been considered an expensive, luxurious fabric reserved for high quality garments. Nowadays, there is a great variety of cheaper silks both dyed and printed originating primarily from Japan.

Artificial or Rayon Silk: material made from viscose.

Ordinary Silk: fabric generally originating from Chinese silkworm cultivation.

Wild Silk: Wild silks are more irregular than ordinary silks; they are used for dresses and blouses, as well as furnishing fabrics.

Tussah: Indian fabric obtained from wild silk worms living in tropical forests. Fibre is naturally golden as the caterpillars eat the bark from tannin-rich trees.

Dupion Silk: a lustrous silk woven from two different coloured threads which shimmer in the light. It is an irregular rough silk reeled from double cocoons or cocoons spun side by side.

Noil or Bourette: this is silk obtained from the crushed pupa left behind after making the higher quality yarns.

Vegetable Silk: material made by weaving herbaceous plants.

Blended Silks:

Silk And Cotton: which looks like silk but has the texture of the second; used for dresses and blouses.

Silk and Wool: by adding wool this blend has all the attributes of warmth and strength yet becomes smoother and silkier due to the blending. Used for suits and jackets.

Silk and Linen:

the silk softens the linen making this fabric suitable for suits, skirts, dresses and trousers.

TAFFETAS

A crisp, rustling, lustrous evening fabric often woven with plaids or shot warp and weft effect. Plain silk weave fabric which derives its name from the Persian word *taftah* meaning 'woven'.

TARTAN

This is a generic term for any fabric which has coloured warps and wefts creating a check pattern, regardless of the material. The kilts belonging to the different Scottish clans each have their own specific pattern, colour or type of check. Tartans, whether they are in cotton or synthetic fibres, are used for unisex clothing, accessories and linings.

TENNIS STRIPES

Fabric with vertical stripes similar to *milleraies* but more spaced apart - can be woven or printed. These stripes are most commonly found woollen flannel fabrics used in suit manufacture.

TOILE

This term has several meanings.
It is one of the three basic weaves - the simplest and oldest one made from linen, cotton or hemp threads. Its weft passes alternatively under and over a warp thread which makes the right side and the reverse identical. The plain weave fabric is gen-

erally light or of medium weight.

This term also applies to a light muslin used for a prototype or test-garment on the dress form.

TULLE

Originating from a town in the department of the Corrèze in France. Light net-type fabric produced using a specific technique and machine with a 'tulle' bobbin which gives the fabric a polygonal, or diagonal, structure. It is normally superimposed onto the another material or used on its own for blouses, dresses and tutus.

TWEED

Scottish woollen material which derives its name from the River Tweed on the borders of Scotland and England. In its classic form (speckled effect) or modern (more colour weave effects and patterns), this material is ideal for the winter. It is used for suits (classic tweed) and jackets or trousers (modern tweed).

TWILL

A reversible woollen fabric with dense threads of twill weave. The relief is reminiscent of the diagonal wales on the face of gabardine, denim, Tricotine (cavalry twill) etc. However, it is less pronounced. It is used for suits and jackets, or where the linings are made with viscose filaments. It is also a term to describe one of the three types of fundamental weaves where the warp threads intersect the wefts producing a fabric with slanting ribs having a right side and a reverse, like denim or gabardine. Used most frequently for coats and suits.

VELVET

This word comes from the Latin *villosus*, which means 'hairy', describes materials made from eastern techniques which give them their luxurious, downy texture. It is dense with a short, closely woven cut pile and is made with two warps: the first for the background, the second for the pile. It can be made in a variety of materials: silk, wool, cotton, viscose, synthetic fibres etc.

Panne Velvet: although generally made from silk, it can be made from synthetic fibres which are woven or knitted. It has a type of finish which gives a shiny, moiré aspect to the fabric. It is light and is used for evening dresses and lingerie.

Corduroy: woven ribbed fabric, where the pile is smooth in only one direction. Supple, comfortable and durable. Used for trousers and jackets.

Cotton Velvet: velvet fabric with a regular 'down' on the right side with the pile being smooth in one direction. Used for evening dresses and furnishing fabrics.

Towelling Velvet: fabric with circular loops on one side with the reverse being smooth.

Crushed Velvet: fabric with crumpled and shimmering aspect made from small tendril-like threads. Used for dresses normally.

VELVET FELT
Very soft, dense, plush fabric.

VENITIAN
The woollen threads are combed to give a luxurious sateen woven wool fabric used for suits and coats.

VISCOSE
This term describes a fabric, as well as a textile manufacturing process. It is a manufactured fibre made of regenerated cellulose (see Cellulose) which is made up in many woven or knitted forms and weights, both mat and shiny. It is soft, absorbent and drapes well, making it an ideal material for dresses and skirts.

VOILE
Plain weave cloth made from cotton, wool or silk, originating from India. It is a lightweight, sheer fabric, coloured or printed and is often used for dresses, camisoles as well as furnishing fabrics such as curtains, net curtains etc.

VYELLA
This is a registered trademark fabric of brushed wool or cotton which can be coloured by weaving or printing. It is used for medium weight winter wear and school uniforms, as well as sheets and nightclothes.

WAX FABRIC
The English imported this technique from Africa (see Bazins). It is used nowadays for the manufacture of the African fabrics (see Pagnes) and the high-quality bazins which are brighter and silkier. This fabric is a printed cotton where the colour is applied with a wax (inspired by batik painting). It is a light, brightly coloured fabric which is used in the manufacture of summer clothing or pagnes.

WAXED
Cotton fabric which has been coated with an oil, or wax, to render the material waterproof. French fishermen from Brittany are famous for their yellow-oilskin dungarees, hat and windcheaters, as is the brand Barbour for its three-quarter length hunter's jackets. Oilskins are used for outdoor waterproof clothing, mainly jackets.

WHIPCORD
This material was originally made from wool has an oblique ribbed texture. Nowadays, the term generally applies to all twill woven fabrics with a diagonal or relief. Its dense texture means it is ideal for suits and jackets.

WINCYETTE
A brushed cotton used for pyjamas and children's wear.

WOOL
Natural fibre obtained from sheep and goats (and certain rabbits in the case of angora). There are a great many variations depending on the different breeds. The texture and weaving of the wool varies also. Generally the wool is mixed between sheep and other ovines and it is warm, absorbent and pleasant to touch. Used for coats, suits, jumpers and furnishing fabrics.

WORSTED
Durable woollen fabric, whose production turned around the fortunes of Bradford in Yorkshire during the Industrial Revolution. It is mainly used for men's suits.

WOVEN CANVAS
Linen or starched cotton or where an adhesive coating has been applied. Mainly used for men's clothing.

YARNS
There are three main types of yarns/plies for weaving and knitting:

Cabled Yarn: a yarn formed by twisting together two or more plied yarns.

Twisted Yarn: assembling of single threads by inverse twisting.

Marl Thread: two different coloured single strands of yarn spun together. This mottled effect is often seen in sweaters.

MACHINES

There are six categories of sewing machines.

CANON MACHINE

This resembles the tubular machine closely however, it is perpendicular to the working bench. It has automatic systems for buttonholes and buttons, as well as being able to do straight and chain stitch.

DOUBLE-NEEDLED MACHINE (with movable arms)

This machine does not have a flat-bed, instead it has a second arm which forms a U at the back of the machine just before its head. This machine facilitates the closing of tubular pieces with turned-up edges or seams such as jeans or shirt sleeves. It can also do straight stitch and chain stitch.

FIVE THREAD SERGER OR OVERLOCKER MACHINE

This machine has 2, 4 or 5 threads for over-locking or over-sewing raw edges of a garment to prevent them fraying. It is capable of great speeds enabling stitching, over-locking and edging simultaneously. It is also capable of doing chain stitch and over-locking.

FLAT BED MACHINE

This machine has one or two needles. Fitted onto an arm, of which there are three sizes depending on the size of the piece to be sewn, it is the oldest and most widespread of sewing machines. Certain flat bed machines have a double or triple feed allowing materials such as leather or denim to be successfully worked. Straight stitch and chain stitch are able to be done with this type of machine.

FIVE THREAD SERGER OR OVERLOCKER MACHINE

This machine has 2, 4 or 5 threads for over-locking or over-sewing raw edges of a garment to prevent them fraying. It is capable of great speeds enabling stitching, over-locking and edging simultaneously. It is also capable of doing chain stitch and over-locking.

TUBULAR OR CIRCULAR MACHINE

This has an arm, like the flat-bed machine, but instead of a bed the material surrounds a tube. Trouser-legs and sleeves are made using this type of machine. It is also capable of doing straight stitch and chain stitch.

SPECIALIST MACHINES

INVISIBLE STITCH MACHINE

This machine has a floating needle (straight with two points), making invisible or blind stitches either side of the material.

INVISIBLE STITCHING MACHINE

Most often tubular in shape, it has a curved needle: when doing a chain stitch, the thread does not go right through the material. Instead it goes into the centre coming out again through the top, where it entered. This machine is used for hemlines and stiffenings.

LOCK-STITCH MACHINE

This makes a chain stitch with one single thread according to normal knitting principles. It is used for making collars, sleeves and cuffs. Its lateral arm, placed under the head, allows for hook and needle movements to be printed.

GLOSSARY

ALL-OVER (MOTIF)
Pattern, or motif, which repeats horizontally as well as vertically, i.e. spots. It is distinguished from the placed motif, which is a single motif, and the repeat pattern, which is repeated in one direction only (such as that of Toile de Jouy).

ALLOWANCE
Extra fabric added to: a seam line, a garment for ease of movement, or for pleats and gathers.

APPLIQUÉ
An element which is stuck or sewn on, like an emblem for example. Or, a decorative patch of fabric sewn or stuck onto another.

ARTISTIC DIRECTOR or CREATIVE DIRECTOR
Person who defines the brand's image and collections. He/she decides which products will be included in the collection.

ASSEMBLE
To sew together the different pieces of a model, or item. Or in lace making, the assembling together of the different pattern elements, such as flowers, leaves etc. to make a flower.

AWL
Sharp pointed tool for making holes in patterns and leather.

BASTING
Temporary stitching, also called tacking, used to hold fabrics together for fittings and before machining.

BIAS
The diagonal line at 45° to the straight and crosswise grain of the fabric. Bias binding is a tape cut 'on the bias'. It has pressed, folded edges and has more give than flat woven tape. Ideal for hemming and seaming.

BONING
Originally made from whale bones, they were used for reinforcing clothes such as corsets, tutus, shirt collar corners. Nowadays, plastic or metal stiffeners are used.

BOOKING
When preparing for a fashion show, or photo shoot, a model, photographer, make-up artist, and hairdresser are signed up to create the team for the presentation.

BOUTIQUE
A shop and its shop window promote the brand's image, and/or the designers and artistic directors who have often styled the interior décor themselves.

BRAINSTORMING
Meeting of colleagues during which different ideas and concepts are exchanged and discussed.

BRANDING
Consumers' desire to buy internationally recognised brand products or ethos.

BREAK LINE
Fold line of a collar lapel, or an ironed fold of a trouser leg or pleat.

BUTTON STAND
Piece of supplementary fabric added to a garment where a fastener or button is to be added, i.e. at the base of a collar.

BUYER
Person responsible for buying, and planning orders, in the buying office of a shop or department store.

BUYING OFFICE (see Buyer)
The department responsible within a store, or an independent body who arrange to buy for chains and boutiques, especially from overseas suppliers.

CAD/CAM
Computer-Aided Design/Computer-Aided Manufacture.

CASTING
Choice of models for a fashion show or a photo shoot.

CLASSIC OR STAPLE GARMENT
Wardrobe item which is easy to wear/everyday use.

COLLAR STAND
The under-collar, before the 'fall' or fold-back of a collar, often reinforced and buttoned on a shirt.

COLLECTION COORDINATOR
Person responsible for the development and organisation of a collection, in the design studio.

COLLECTION PLAN
Plan itemising the number of fabrics and items necessary for the different products: coats, jackets, skits, trousers, dresses, tops, etc. It defines the structure of a collection and can be presented either by a written document, or presentation boards with sketches detailing the fabrics organised by product type.

COLOUR CHART
Collection of several referenced colours facilitating choice. Pantone being the registered trademark company.

COLOUR HARMONIES
Classification of the colour tones used in a colour way, or the balance of the chosen colours in the given proportions of a collection.

COLOUR PALETTE
Presentation of a large number of colours from which a choice will be made to narrow down the finished colour range, or gamut, for the collection.

COLOURWAY
The name given to a limited range of colours chosen for a style or collection. It is also used for the choice of colours available for a fabric (knitwear, print, Jacquard etc.).

CONVERTER

A manufacturer who treats raw fibres making them into a fabric or converts greige goods (pronounced grey) into fabrics. Different processes are used for different raw products to improve their quality: wool is felted, fabric is mercerised to give it a shiny appearance, waterproofing, etc.

CONTOUR MASTER

Curved ruler used by pattern makers.

COUTURIER

This was a French term used in the 1960s and 1970s to describe the fashion designer of a brand in reference to the *haute couture* sector. Nowadays the term 'artistic director' is used

CREATOR

Term used in the 1980s to describe a designer.

CROQUIS

A line drawing or sketch made by the designer to illustrate a garment or a painted out design for a printed fabric. It shows the lines of the style, garment look or pattern.

CUT AND SEWN

Term used to describe products which are made from industrially knitted materials (jerseys) made on a roll or cylinder.

CROTCH OR CRUTCH

Seam between the legs of a pair of trousers, shorts, Bermudas or culottes

CUSTOM TAILORED/BESPOKE

Individual made to measure tailoring for suits.

CUT

Assembly lines of a garment, as with the Princess lines in a dress and straps in the case of a top.

CUTTING

Production stage where the different pieces of the garment are cut from the fabric.

CUTTING or LAY PLAN

Plan for the pattern pieces to be cut according to the width and type of material.

DART

A stitched down fold, tapering at one or both ends, to allow the fabric to follow the shape of the body.

DECOLLETÉ

Low neckline, without a collar (boat, V-neck etc.).

DECONSTRUCTION

A style of designing originating with Belgian designers where the garments were left rough or unfinished, or revealing construction details.

DESIGN CONSULTANTS OR STYLE BUREAU

Outside agency which proposes to its clients (brands, industry, distributors or fashion show organisers) advice on trends, design and product research.

DESIGNER

General term used to describe a fashion designer, as well as any one working in the design field.

DETAILS

Pieces or finishes of a garment such as pockets etc.

DIFFUSION LINE

A secondary, usually lower-priced garment line that allows consumers, on a budget, to buy the designer 'look' and for the manufacture to maximise sales.

DRAPING

In the fashion world this refers to the fitting of a fabric onto a dress form to make the *toile* or sample garment. The term 'draped' refers to giving volume to a fabric.

DRESS FORM OR STAND

Toiliste or pattern cutter's work tool, which is the body form of a torso of average size, i.e. 10 (38), usually on a stand which rotates to help the pattern cutter make the toile and work on the garment.

EASE

Similar to allowance i.e. extra fabric to allow for loose fit and comfort.

EDGE TO EDGE

Two pieces of a garment which join, without crossing, such as a zip fastening.

EMPIRE LINE

Dress with a short bodice, usually with a seam or drawstring under the bust.

FACING

Interior of a garment made in the same fabric as the garment itself. It is attached to a lining, if there is one, finishing off the piece properly.

FALL OF A GARMENT

The look of a garment which is determined by the cut and mastering volume. There are certain rules which need to be adhered to if a garment is to have a good fall.

FASHION

Term used to describe the influence of one season, although a trend, or fashion, can last a decade.

FASHION CULTURE

Collection of signs, codes, language, images and reference which define the world of fashion.

FASHION CYCLE

The time necessary to develop a collection, including planning, designing, making and marketing, in relation to a determined market. The cycle will vary according to the different market.

FASHION ILLUSTRATION OR PLATE
Stylised design of the silhouette volume used to express the idea of a garment.

FASHION STYLIST
Person responsible for creating the 'look' for a shoot, by coordinating the fabrics and accessories.

FEELER or SWATCH
A sample of fabric offered by salesmen to help the designer make a choice of material or colour ways.

FIT MODEL
A live model who is used as the company's standard sizing sample for the fittings.

FITTING
Work session where the modeller and the designer work together to confirm the fit and details of a garment. This fitting is carried out using half the *toile* or the entire one, on the dress form or on a 'fit model'. Normally this requires three fittings to arrive at a successful conclusion.

FLARED
To cut a garment on the bias to obtain a trapeze, or flared, effect such as pagoda sleeves, bell-bottomed trousers, A-line skirts, skirts with godet inset, Flapper dresses or the Redingote jacket.

FLAT COLOUR
Application of a colour in a way that the surface is painted smooth and uniformly where no paintbrush, or felt pen mark, is visible.

FLAT PATTERN DRAFTING (see Lay plan)
Precision drawing that requires accurate measurements and use of proportion to make a lay plan.

FOUR-COLOUR PRINTING
The three primary colours (red, blue and yellow) then the black.

FRENCH CURVE
Pattern cutting tool with a 'golden mean' to aid the drafting of tight and open curves.

FROG FASTENINGS
Trimming loops or straps used as garment fastenings.

GATHERS
Fabric which is drawn up for ease or fullness on a double line of stitches. Used to give volume to the head of a sleeve, skirt on a dress or to drape a jersey material.

GODET
A triangular piece of fabric inserted into the bias, or hem, of a skirt to give it flare and movement.

GRADING
Operation which consists of sizing a pattern up or down the standard measurement fitting.

GROSGRAIN
A broad, stiff ribbon with striped relief used for waistbands and hat trimmings.

GUSSET
Triangular or lozenge-shaped piece of material inset into another piece of fabric for ease of movement or comfort. It can be added to sleeves, in the case of a kimono or underarm, or into the crotch of a pair of trousers.

HABERDASHERY
General term for garment trimmings including needles, threads, ribbons, buttons, fasteners etc.

HAUTE COUTURE
French term used for the highest quality of bespoke dressmaking. Designers will use specific accessory metiers such as feather makers, jewellers, embroiderers, furriers etc. to embellish their designs. Designers cannot call themselves *haute couture* unless they have been passed by the Chambre Syndicale de la Fédération Française de la Couture.

HEAT-FUSIBLE
With the aid of a press, the glue which is present on a cloth such as an interfacing is melted. This gives a type of reinforcement to the material in areas such as collars, cuffs and facings.

INSET
A piece of fabric or trimming used decoratively in a seam.

LACING
Two edges with eyelets and ties, or laces that can be adjusted to vary fits. Used for fastening garments or decorative details.

LAIZE
Direction of the width of a fabric.

LAMINATE
To coat, glue or heat-bond two fabrics together.

LAPEL SEAM
Interior seam of a suit jacket collar, at the point where the collar and the lapel meet.

LICENCE
Contract giving authorisation to use a brand, logo, type of product or a concept by a third party in exchange for royalty payments.

LINE
Schematic shape of a garment, or a range of products developed around the same theme.

LUREX
Metallic thread used either pure, or mixed, of coloured metal – gold, silver, platinum, copper etc. but can also be red, blue, green etc.

LUXURY *PRÊT-À-PORTER*
Term used to describe the top end of *prêt-à-porter* goods in general.

MAQUETTE
Mock-up made to illustrate a project either, on the flat, or by volume: can be a drawing for a textile print, a model for some jewellery, or the heel of a shoe. The term maquette is also used for the visual identity of a catalogue or magazine; it includes the page layout, choice of typeface and visuals.

MARKET
Group of people established according to geographical criteria, consisting of different types of consumers having specific commercial constraints.

MARKETING DEPARTMENT
Department or office dealing with a company's promotion and coordination thereof.

MERCHANDISING
Term used to denote all aspects of optimising commercial results.

MIX AND MATCH
Term used to describe garments which are mixed, assortment of, organised and coordinated.

MODELLING
Term used in the fashion world to denote the method of construction of the garment: it consists of working from a flat drawing in the first instance, to give a garment volume according to the different methods of construction, i.e. flat pattern-drafting or draping.

MOODBOARD
A presentation board which gives the overall concept and direction of the design collection, including photos, fabric swatches, colours and sketches.

MUSIC PRODUCER/SOUND ENGINEER
Person responsible for the research and soundtracks used in a fashion show, publicity film, educational video.

NOTCH
Marks cut into the seam allowances of patterns, or fabrics, to indicate sewing positions and match balance points made by a tool called a pattern notcher. They can also be used around necklines and armholes to make the curves more rounded and supple.

PASSEMENTERIES
Finishing details done using thread used to embellish a garment (shoulder pads, emblems, braids etc.).

PATTERN-DRAFTING, CUTTING AND MAKING
The drawing out of a flat pattern, made from card or paper, using measurements or through the use of block templates. Comprising all the pieces necessary for a garment

PATTERN HOOK
Commercial patterns are usually stored by hanging onto a metal hook, rather than folding.

PEPLUM
Bottom part of a jacket which descends from the waist to hip level.

PERSONAL SHOPPER
Person responsible for selecting products for a particular client who does not have the time to do the research themselves.

PINBOARD
Board covered with fine pins on which smooth or ribbed velvet is placed so that the pile is not squashed.

PINKING SHEARS
Serrated shears used to cut fabric or seam allowances to prevent fraying.

PIPING
Strip of fabric added to the slit of a pocket or buttonhole, or run into a seam to bind or decorate the edge.

PLEATS
Pleats can be made by regular manipulation of a fabric into a yoke or waistband, or by an industrial steaming process. There are many different types, i.e. box, flat, kick, inverted, knife etc. There are some fabrics which are made up of a series of pleated fabrics such as Fortuny and Issey Miyake's pleated fabrics.

PR and EVENTS ORGANISER
Office or department which is responsible for the organisation of the fashion shows, product launches, boutique openings etc.

PRESS OFFICER
Person responsible for the public relations of a brand or company.

PRINCESS LINE
A slim dress, or bodice shape, using only vertical seam lines starting at the armhole.

RAGLAN SLEEVE
Sleeve made in two pieces with a seam line running down the top of the sleeve from the neckline to the bottom. Gives the shoulder a more or less rounded effect.

RESEARCH DEPARTMENT
Where the prototypes are developed and technical services are offered, such as regulating and grading the patterns, as well as launching the collection.

RETRO PLANNING
Planning a work schedule working backwards, i.e. from the date of the presentation to the finished product to the date of the fashion show etc.

ROUGHS

Quick first stage drawings or sketches, usually made in pencil and without extraneous detail, which illustrate the idea.

RUCHED

Slightly puckered folds of ruched material are almost a cross between a fold and a dart

SAMPLE

First model of a garment, made in the definitive fabric or, one as close as possible, which tests whether the garment will be kept in the collection or not. It is rare that the first prototype is able to be shown to sales or marketing teams – normally several prototypes are made.

SAMPLE LENGTH

Small amount of fabric from which the prototype is cut.

SATURATED (COLOUR)

Colour which has been pushed to its maximum intensity.

SCENE COSTUME

Garment created for a piece of theatre, ballet, concert or opera.

SELVEDGE/SELVAGE

The finished lengthwise woven edge that binds the width of a fabric preventing fraying.

SHIRT SLEEVE

Sleeve with buttoned cuff.

SHOOT

Photo session.

SHOULDER PAD

Piece of padding or foam added to a shoulder to support the hang of a jacket or coat. There are several different types: tailored shoulder pad, raglan, half-raglan etc.

SHOULDER ROLL

Either a pre-formed piece of foam or material, shaped and placed in a garment to reinforce and form the shoulder shape.

SHOWROOM

Space where the collections are presented to the press and buyers.

SILHOUETTE

General look of a person. In the fashion world , it Is also the collection of elements which make up an outfit, reduced to basic geometric description e.g. boxy, A-line, figure-8 etc. and the name given to a fashion show appearance, i.e. silhouette No.1, No. 2 etc.

SMOCKING

Areas of ornamental stitching on a garment which gathers up the cloth tightly in stitches to form a relief.

SOURCING

Research of ideas, suppliers, markets and other useful elements necessary to make a product.

SPECIFICATION SHEET

A design drawing with measurements, manufacturing details, such as trimmings and stitching, as well as front and back views of the garment, which is annexed to the fashion illustration. It also serves as a gauge for pricing the garment.

STIFFENING

Cloth added to the inside of a suit jacket to reinforce the structure.

STORYBOARD

Also known as a theme board, a presentation of the concept for a collection with the breakdown of styles and coordinates.

STRAIGHT GRAIN

Line running parallel to the warp thread of a fabric which gives the garment its balance. It is the direction of the weave of a fabric.

STRIP

Width of fabric between the two selvedge edges.

STUDIO

Work space where the collections are conceived and designed. For photographs, it is the space where atmospheres are created with lighting and décor.

STUDIO DIRECTOR

Person responsible for the design studio. He/she coordinates the workload of each of the designers in relation to the artistic director's instructions.

STYLE DEVELOPMENTS

This involves research from a given idea for different models, volumes, shapes and products.

TAILORED SLEEVE

Sleeve which has a top and an underneath part so that the elbow can be worked. The top of the sleeve is made so that it has a rounded volume giving a particular tailored line to the jacket or coat.

TAILOR'S CHALK

Waxy chalk which is puffed or drawn onto the fabric to mark the positions and guides for the machinists. The chalk is easily removed with steam.

TEMPLATE

Piece of card which guides the machinist when making pockets or collars. It is a pattern piece without the seams.

TEXTURE

A material's structure and consistence.

TICKING

Cotton twill-weave fabric characterised by its dense and strong qualities, used mainly for work clothing and furnishings, notably mattress coverings.

TOILE
Mock up, or draft, of a garment made in a fabric similar to natural-coloured muslin and worked on a dress form.

TONES
All the intermediary colours obtained from a single one.

TREND
A trend lasts a decade, contrary to the fashion world, where it lasts just a season. It is a well-used term in the fashion industry to announce themes and future season ideas.

TREND BOOK AND FORECASTING
Forecasting book which presents all the season's trends concerning colour, fabrics, looks, beauty products and style. Prospective studies are done by a body of people who come together twice a year to summarise and define the broad industry trends for a given market.

TRIMMINGS
A term used for the decorative details on a garment such as, fur on a collar or cuffs of a coat, and for the process of finishing or cutting loose threads.

TURN UP
The underside of a collar when turned up or added cuff at the trouser hem.

VINTAGE
Old garment, representative of an era, conserved in its original state.

WARP and WEFT
Term used by professionals to refer to the direction of the weave. The warp threads of a woven fabric are those which make up the lengthwise grain. The weft threads are placed in by a shuttle, at 90° to the warp, and run from selvedge to selvedge giving the fabric its width.

WEAVE
Method of organisation of a fabric's warp and weft threads. There are three principal arrangements: plain, twill or satin weaves, from which innumerable combinations are derived.

WHIPPING/OVER-SEWING
Finishing stitch on a garment which stops any fraying of the fabric after it is cut. It is commonly used for knitwear and jersey.

WORKROOM/ATELIER
Place where the samples and prototypes are developed and where technicians, such as, toilistes/pattern cutters, machinists and cutters, work.

Flou, Or Dressmaking, Workroom: place where dresses, blouses and unstructured items are developed.

Suit Tailoring Workroom: place where fitted sleeves are made requiring a specific skill as seen in suits, costumes and coats etc.

These are the two types of workshops most commonly encountered in the world of *haute couture*.

Assembly Workroom: this where batch production items are made up.

Cutting Workroom: place where the above are cut.

YOKE
A piece of material used to support a fuller or gathered length, e.g. across the shoulders of a shirt or from the hip line.

ZIG ZAG
Stitch used to bind or finish edges decoratively or where the seam must be allowed to stretch safely, i.e. with knitwear and lingerie.

FASHION DIRECTORY

SHOPS AND SUPPLIERS

FABRICS
France

Bouchara
1-3, rue La Fayette
75009 Paris

Dreyfus
2, rue Charles-Nodier
75018 Paris

Pierre Frey
22, rue Royale
75008 Paris

De Gilles
156, rue de la Roquette
75011 Paris

Huguet et Cie (fils de laine)
36, rue Réaumur
75003 Paris

Dominique Kieffer
8, rue Hérold
75001 Paris

Le Rouvray
3, rue de la Bûcherie
75005 Paris

Marché Carreau du Temple
2, rue Perrée
75003 Paris

Mokuba (rubans, passementerie)
18, rue Montmartre
75001 Paris

Moline Tissus
1, place Saint-Pierre
75018 Paris

Reine
5, place Saint-Pierre
75018 Paris

UK

Borovicks Fabrics Ltd
16 Berwick Street
London W1F 0HP
020 7437 2180
www.borovickfabricsltd.co.uk

Cloth House
47 Berwick Street
London W1F 8SJ
020 7437 5155

Cloth House
98 Berwick Street
London W1F 0QJ
020 7287 1555

Cloth Shop
14 Berwick Street
London W1F 0PP
020 7287 2881

MacCulloch & Wallis
25-26 Dering Street
London W1S 1AT
www.maccullock-wallis.co.uk

Silk Society
44 Berwick Street
London W1F 8SE
020 7287 1881

DRAWING SUPPLIERS

Cass Art
13 Charing Cross Road
London WC2H 0EP
0207930 9940
www.cass-arts.co.uk

L. Cornelissen & Son
105 Great Russell Street
London WC1B 3RY
020 7636 1045
www.cornelissen.com

Cowling & Wilcox
26-28 Broadwick Street
London W1F 8HX
020 7734 9556
www.cowlingandwilcox.com

London Graphic Centre
16-18 Shelton Street
London WC2H 9JL
020 7759 4500
www.londongraphics.co.uk

STUDIO AND BOUTIQUE EQUIPMENT

MacCulloch & Wallis
25-26 Dering Street
London W1S 1AT
www.macculloch-wallis.co.uk

Morplan
56 Great Titchfield Street
London W1W 7DF
020 7636 1887

SUNDRIES

Button Queen
19 Marylebone Lane
London W1U 2NF
020 7935 1505

Cloth House
47 Berwick Street
London W1F 8SJ
020 7437 5155

MacCulloch & Wallis
25-26 Dering Street
London W1S 1AT
www.macculloch-wallis.co.uk

V. V. Rouleaux
54 Sloane Street
London SW1W 8AX
020 7730 3125
www.vvrouleaux.com

V. V. Rouleaux
94 Miller Street
Glasgow G1 1DT
0141 221 2277
www.vvrouleaux.com

USEFUL ADDRESSES

British Fashion Council
5 Portland Place
London W1B 1PW
020 7636 7788

FASHION SCHOOLS

France

Atelier Chardon Savard
BTS Stylisme de mode
15, rue Gambey
75011 Paris

Chambre syndicale de la couture parisienne
Formations aux métiers artistiques
45, rue Saint-Roch
75001 Paris

École C-SIX-DOUZE
École supérieure privée art et design
44 bis, rue Lucien-Sampaix
75010 Paris

École Duperré
BTS Mode-Textile DMA Arts textiles (DSAA Mode et Environnement)
11, rue Dupetit-Thouars
75003 Paris

ENSAAMA Olivier de Serres
BTS Art textile et Impression
63-65, rue Olivier-de-Serres
75015 Paris

ESMOD
École supérieure privée de création de mode
12, rue La Rochefoucauld
75009 Paris

LISAA
13, rue Vaucquelin
75005 Paris

Lycée Auguste Renoir
Arts appliqués (spécialisation industrie de l'habillement, prépa BT)
24, rue Ganneron
75018 Paris

Lycée Choiseul
BTS Arts appliqués stylisme de mode
78, rue des Douets
39095 Tours

Lycée de la mode
BTS Stylisme de mode
20, rue du Carteron
49321 Cholet

Lycée Elisa Lemonnier
20, avenue Armand-Rousseau
75012 Paris

STUDIO Burçu
29, rue des Petites-Écuries
75010 Paris

Belgium

Académie royale des Beaux-Arts d'Anvers
Blindestraat 9
BE-2000 Anvers

Flanders Fashion Institute
Mode Natie
Nationale Straat
Drukkerijstraat
Anvers

Hogeschool Antwerp
Fashion Department
Nationalestraat 28/3
2000 Antwerp (Anvers)

La Cambre
École supérieure d'Arts visuels
21, abbaye de la Cambre
1000 Bruxelles

UK

Central Saint Martin's College of Art and Design
School of Fashion and Textiles
107-109 Charing Cross Road
London WC2H 0DU

Edinburgh College of Art
Lauriston Place
Edinburgh EH3 9DF

Kingston University
School of Fashion
Knights Park
Kingston upon Thames
Surrey KT1 2QJ

London College of Fashion
20 John Princes Street
London W1M 0BJ

Manchester Metropolitan University
Faculty of Art & Design
Ormond Building
Ormond Street
Manchester M15 6BH

Middlesex University
School of Fashion and Textiles
Cat Hill
Barnet
Hertfordshire EN4 8HT

Royal College of Art
(MA course only)
School of Fashion and Textiles
Kensington Gore
London SW7 2EU

University of Brighton
School of Design - Fashion Textiles
Grand Parade, Brighton
East Sussex BN2 2U

University of Newcastle upon Tyne
Department of Fine Art
5 Kensington Terrace
Newcastle upon Tyne NE4 7SA

USA

Parsons School of Design
560 Fashion Avenue
New York, NY 10018

Japan

Bunka Fashion College
3-22-1 Yoyogi Shibuya-Ku Tokyo

Doreme Sugino Gakuen
4-6-19 Oosaki Shibuya-Ku Tokyo

Esmod Japon
3-29-6 Ebisu Shibuya-Ku Tokyo

Mode Gakuen
1-6-2 Nishishinjuku Shibuya-Ku Tokyo

Vantan Design Institute
3-9-4 Ebisu-Minami Shibuya-Ku Tokyo

RECRUITMENT SITES FOR
FASHION PROFESSIONALS

www.abc-luxe.com

www.bethe1.com

www.fashionjob.fr

www.ks-interim.com

www.lejournaldutextile.com

www.modefashion.com

www.modemonline.com

www.profilmode.com

Chantal Baudron
61, boulevard Haussmann
75008 Paris
www.chantal-baudron.fr
Fashion Expert
54, rue du Faubourg-Montmartre
75009 Paris
Tél. : 01 44 63 13 52

Floriane de St-Pierre
134, rue du Faubourg-Saint-Honoré
75008 Paris

Interim Nation
75, boulevard de Picpus
75012 Paris
www.interim-nation.fr
Tél. : 01 43 45 50 00

Janou Parker
4, rue du Faubourg-Saint-Honoré
75008 Paris
Tél : 01.45.23.18.54

Manpower Couture
42, rue Washington
75008 Paris
Tél. : 01 56 59 32 70

Modelor
18-20, rue Daunou
75002 Paris
www.modelor.fr

Proman Paris Saint-Lazare
2, rue de l'Isly
75008 Paris
Tél. : 01 53 42 18 30
www.poman-interim.com

Kate Sasson conseil
21, rue Cambon
75001 Paris
www.katesasson.com

Sterling (Mickaël Boroian)
1, rue François-1er
75008 Paris
Tél : 01.55.73.30.00
Vedior bis couture
120, boulevard Diderot
72012 Paris
Tél. : 01 43 44 32 00

LIBRARIES

Libraries in Paris :

Les Archives de la presse
51, rue des Archives
75003 Paris
Tél. : 01 42 72 93 72

Les Arts décoratifs
63, rue Monceau
75008 Paris
Tél. : 01 53 89 06 40

Bibliothèque des Arts décoratifs
107, rue de Rivoli
75001 Paris
Tél. : 01 44 55 57 50

Bibliothèque municipale de la Ville de Paris
Bibliothèque Forney et arts graphiques
- Hôtel de Sens
1, rue du Figuier
75004 Paris
Tél. : 01 42 78 14 60

Bibliothèque nationale de France
Bibliothèque François-Mitterrand
11, quai François-Mauriac
75013 Paris

Bibliothèque Publique d'Information
- Centre Georges-Pompidou
19, rue Beaubourg
75004 Paris
Tél. : 01 44 78 12 33

Musée Galliera - musée de la Mode de la Ville
de Paris
Centre de documentation - bibliothèque
10, avenue Pierre-1er-de-Serbie
75115 Paris
Tél. : 01 56 52 86 00

MUSEUMS

France:

Centre Georges-Pompidou
19, rue Beaubourg
75004 Paris

Fondation Cartier
261, boulevard Raspail
75014 Paris

Musée des Arts décoratifs
107, rue de Rivoli
75001 Paris

Musée du Costume de la Ville de Paris
14, avenue de New York
75016 Paris

Musée Galliera
10, avenue Pierre-Ier-de-Serbie
75016 Paris

Musée de l'Impression sur étoffes
14, rue Jean-Jacques-Henner
BP1468
68072 Mulhouse Cedex

Musée de la Mode de Marseille
11, La Canebière
13001 Marseille

Musée de la Mode et du Textile
107, rue de Rivoli
75001 Paris

Musée des Tissus et des Arts décoratifs
34, rue de la Charité
69002 Lyon

Palais de Tokyo
2, rue de la Manutention
75116 Paris

UK

Design Museum
Shad Thames,
London SE1 2YD
020 7403 6933

Fashion Museum
Assembly Rooms
Bennett Street
Bath
BA1 2QH
Tel: +44 (0) 1225 477173

Fashion and Textile Museum
83 Bermondsey Street
London
SE1 3XF

T: 020 7407 8664

National Museum of Costume
Shambellie House
New Abbey
Dumfriesshire
Scotland
DG2 8HQ
Tel: 01387 850 37

National Wool Museum
Dre-Fach Felindre
near Newcastle Emlyn
Llandysul
Carmarthenshire
Wales
SA44 5UP
(01559) 370929

Victora & Albert Museum
Cromwell Road
London SW7 2RL
+44 (0)20 7942 2000

PRINCIPAL TRADE FAIRS

Accessories
Modamont (Paris)
Première classe

Leather
Anteprima (Milan)
Le cuir à Paris
Linea Pelle (accessoires et prêt-à-porter)
Salon du cuir

Yarn
Expofil (Paris) : septembre et mars
Indigo

Knitwear
Expofil (Paris)
Moda In (Milan)
Pitti Filatil (Florence)

Prêt-à-porter
Atmosphère (Hotel St James)
Tranoï
Who's next

Finished products
Intersélection

Fabrics
Moda In (Milan)
Première Vision (Paris) : septembre et mars
Texworld (Paris)
Tissu Premier (Lille) : janvier

appendices

BIBLIOGRAPHY

Books

Big Active, *Head, Heart & Hips – The Seductive World of Big Active*, Berlin, Die Gelstalten Verlag, Edition, 2004.

Susanna Anna, Eva Gronback, Miriam Matsuszkiewicz, *The Fashion Generation*, New York, Hatje Cantz Publishers, 2006.

Maggy Baum, Chantal Boyeldieu, *Dictionnaire des textiles*, Paris, Éditions de l'industrie textile, 2003.

George Beylerian, Andrew Dent, *Material connexion – The global resource of new and innovative materials for architects, artists and designers*, New York, John Wiley & Sons Editions, 2005.

François Boucher, *Histoire du costume en Occident de l'Antiquité à nos jours*, Paris, Flammarion, 1983.

David Bowie, Karl Lagerfeld, Mario Testino, *Dreaming in Print : a Decade of Visionnaire*, New York, Éditions 7L (Steidl), 2002.

Collectif, *Beyond Desire*, New York, Ludion, 2005.

Collectif, *Embroidery*, New York, Damiani, 2006.

Collectif, *Fabrica 10 – From chaos to order and back*, Milan, Electa s.p.a., 2004.

Collectif, *Technologie du vêtement*, Québec, Guérin, 1999.

Collectif, *Total Living*, New York, Charta, 2002.

Collectif, *Uniform : Order and Disorder*, New York, Charta, 2001.

Collectif, *Modemuseum/The Fashion Museum*, New York, Ludion, 2003 .

Collectif, *Shopping*, New York, Hatje Cantz Publishers, 2003.

Luc Dericke, Sandra Van De Veire, *Belgian Fashion Design*, New York, Ludion, 1999.

Dictionnaire international de la mode, Paris, Éditions du Regard, 1994-2004.

Maria Luisa Frisa, Stefano Tonchi, *Excess : Fashion and the Underground in the 80s*, New York, Charta / Fondazione Pitti Immagine Discovery, 2004.

Christine Garaud, Bernadette Sautreuil, *Technologie des tissus*, Paris, André Casteilla, 1984.

Antoine Kruk, *Shibuya Soul*, Paris, Archimbaud, 2006.

Pierre Hirsch, *Lexique textile, français – British*, Metz, Librairie de l'industrie textile, 1994.

Pierre Hirsch, *Textile glossary, anglais – français*, Metz, Librairie de l'industrie textile, 1994.

Sue Jenkyn Jones, *Le Stylisme, guide des métiers*, Paris, Pyramid ntcv, 2005.

Dorling Kindersley, *Le Grand Livre de la couture*, Paris, Hachette, 1997.

Didier Ludot, *La Petite Robe noire*, Paris, Assouline, 2001.

Stéphane Marais, *Beauty Flash*, Paris, 7L Steidl, 2001.

Isaac Mizrahi, *The Adventures of Sandee the Supermodel*, New York, S&S Editions Comic Book Series, 1997.

Ludovico Pratesi, Vichy Hassan, Gianluca Lo Vetro, *Artenergie*, New York, Charta, 1998.

András Szunyoghy et György Fehér, *Anatomie humaine à l'usage des artistes*, Cologne, Köneman, 2000.

Françoise Tellier-Loumagne, *Mailles, les mouvements du fil*, Genève, Minerva, 2003.

Heidemaria Tengler-Stadelmaier, *La Couture pratique, Hoenheim*, V. A. Burda, 2002.

Walter Van Beirendonck, *Mode 2001 : Landed-Geland Part I*, New York, Merz, 2002.

Walter Van Beirendonck, *Mode 2001 : Landed-Geland Part II*, New York, Merz, 2002.

Nadine Vasseur, *Les Plis*, Paris, Le Seuil, 2002.

Veerle Windels, *Young Belgian Fashion Design*, New York, Ludion, 2001.

Fashion trade publications

Bloom

California Apparel News

Daily News Record (DNR)

Fashion Daily News

Fashion Reporter

Journal du textile

Selvedge

Tank

Texnews (www.texnews.fr)

Textile View

Tobe Report

View textile

Womens Wear Daily (WWD)

Fashion magazines

Another magazine (British)

Another man (mode homme – British)

Arena homme + (mode homme – British)

Biba (French)

Citizen K (French)

Collezioni (Italian)

Crash (French)

Deutsch (German)

Doingbird (Australian)

Elle (international)

Figaro Madame (French)

Glamour (international)

GQ (mode homme – international)

Harper's Bazaar (international)

ID (British)

Jalouse (French)

Marie Claire (international)

Milk (mode enfant – French)

Muteen (French)

Neo2 (Spanish)

Numéro (French)

Nylon (American)

L'Officiel (French)

Oyster (Australian)

Pop (British)

Purple (French)

Quest (German)

Self-Service (French)

Sleek (German)

Stilleto (French)

Tank (British)

Ten (British)

Ten men (version homme – British)

L'Uomo Vogue (mode homme – Italian)

V (American)

V men (version homme – American)

20 ans (French)

Visionaire (American)

Vogue (international)

W (American)

Wad (French)

Zoo (German)

FILMOGRAPHY

Amadeus
Milos Foreman, 1984
Inspirational film for XVIII century costumes.

American Gigolo
Paul Schrader, 1980
With Richard Gere playing the role of a high-class gigolo dressed in Armani.

Le Bal
Ettore Scola, 1983
Evolution of fashion from the 1920s to 1950s portrayed in the setting of a ballroom.

Barbarella
Roger Vadim, 1967
Futuristic film with Jane Fonda and costumes by Paco Rabanne.

Barry Lyndon
Stanley Kubrick, 1975
Inspirational film for XVIII century costumes.

Belle de Jour
Luis Bunuel, 1967
Catherine Deneuve is dressed by Yves Saint Laurent.

Bilitis
David Hamilton, 1977
Soft eroticism and romance.

Blade Runner
Ridley Scott, 1982
Science-fiction film, with costumes from the 1940s with a touch of futurism.

Blow up
Michelangelo Antonioni, 1966
Swinging London in the 1960s with the Mary Quant style; the world of a fashion photographer with Veruschka and Jane Birkin.

Blue Angel
Joseph von Sternberg, 1930
Germany in the 1920s, with Marlène Dietrich in her famous theatre costume.

Bonnie and Clyde
Arthur Penn, 1967
American fashion of the 1930s with Faye Dunaway and Warren Beatty.

Breakfast at Tiffany's
Blake Edwards, 1961
The elegance and style of Audrey Hepburn.

Breathless
Jean-Luc Goddard 1959
Jean Seberg: her style, hair and tomboy-look.

Ciao! Manhattan
Andy Warhol, 1972
Edie Sedgwick, one of Andy Warhol's muses icon of the 1970s in New York.

Clockwork Orange
Stanley Kubrick, 1971
1960s style and the influence of the boy look on men's fashion up to today.

The Cook, the Thief, his wife and her lover
Peter Greenaway, 1988
Very stylised film with costumes by Jean-Paul Gaultier.

Desperately Seeking Susan
Susan Seidelman, 1985
The Madonna look of the 1980s.

The Devil wears Prada
David Frankel, 2006
Film about the life of a fashion editor in New York.

La Dolce Vita
Frederico Fellini, 1960
Cult film with Anita Ekberg about Italian society in the 1950s and 60s

Donkey Skin
Jacques Demy, 1970
Princess dresses worn by Catherine Deneuve.

Dracula
Francis Ford Coppola, 1992
Dandy look at the end of the XIX century.

Dune
David Lynch, 1984
Science fiction film, futuristic look and original costumes by Bob Ringwood.

Easy Rider
Dennis Hopper, 1968
Hippy-look and biker's dress in the 1960s and 70s with Dennis Hopper, Jack Nicholson and Peter Fonda.

The Eyes of Laura Mars
Irvin Kershner, 1978
Suspense film around a fashion photographer played by Faye Dunaway with original photos by Helmut Newton.

Fahrenheit 451
François Truffaut, 1966
An imagined futuristic film in the 1960s.

The Fifth Element
Luc Besson, 1997
Science fiction film with Mila Jovovich in Jean-Paul Gaultier's costumes.

Flash Dance
Adrian Lyne, 1983
Explosion of Lycra body-stockings and dance wear.

Funny Face
Stanley Donen, 1957
Audrey Hepburn is dressed by Hubert de Givenchy

Gilda
Charles Vidor, 1946
With Rita Hayworth; Hollywood glamour style in 1940s.

The Girl with the Pearl Earring
Peter Webber, 2004
Historical film inspired by a Vermeer painting.

Grease
Randal Kleiser, 1978
School girl Olivia Newton-John transforms herself into a femme fatale at the end of the 1950s.

The Great Gatsby
Jack Clayton, 1974
Life in the 1930s in America's high-bourgeois society.

The Great Rock 'n Roll Swindle
Julien Temple 1980
Punk film.

Hair
Milos Forman, 1979
Film about the hippy movement.

In the Mood for Love
Wong Kar Wai, 2000
Hongkong in the 1950s – very stylised.

Jules et Jim
François Truffaut, 1962
Jeanne Moreau in the role of a free-spirited women in 1910.

Kids
Larry Clark, 1995
Film about the youth culture in New York in the 1990s.

Kika
Pedro Almodovar, 1993
Costumes by Jean-Paul Gaultier.

Last Year in Marienbad
Alain Resnais, 1961
This film presents the sumptuous years of the 1950s with Delphine Seyrig wearing a Chanel dress.

Liquid Sky
Slava Tsukerman, 1982
Underground cult film of the New Wave era.

Lolita
Stanley Kubrick, 1962
Lolita fashion – fashion subculture in Japan, primarily influenced by Victorian children's clothes as well as costumes from the Rococo period.

Lucifer Rising, Invocation of my demon Brother, Scorpio Rising, Inauguration of the pleasure Dome....
Kenneth Anger, 1970-81, 1969, 1963, 1954
A source of multiple inspiration, in particular, the underground world.

Mad Max I, II and III
George Miller, 1979, 1981, 1985
Science fiction films with futuristic warriors.

Marie Antoinette
Sofia Coppola, 2005
Sumptuous staging of a historical film.

Matrix, Matrix Reloaded, Matrix Revolutions
Andy and Larry Wachowski, 1999, 2003, 2003
Futuristic black film somewhere between gothic and dandy costumes.

Metropolis
Fritz Lang, 1925
Cult science-fiction film set in the 1920s.

Model
Frederick Wiseman, 1980
Modelling agency in New York in the 1970s.

Morocco
Josef von Sternberg, 1930
Marlène Dietrich in a smoking jacket.

Notebook on Cities and Clothes
Wim Wenders, 1989
Film about the designer Yohji Yamamoto.

Pandora's Box
Georg Wilhelm Pabst, 1929
Louise Brooks and her famous 'bob' cut and style.

Performance
Donald Cammell and Nicholas Roeg, 1970
Swinging London with Mick Jagger and Anita Pallenberg dressed by Ossie Clark.

Pret-a-porter
Robert Altman, 1994
Film presenting the world of the Parisian fashion scene with fashion shows by Christian Lacroix and Jean-Paul Gaultier.

Quadrophenia
Franc Roddam, 1979
Film about the mods and rockers in the 1960s featuring Sting.

Reservoir Dogs
Quentin Tarantino, 1992
Black suits, white shirts and thin black ties....
Rize
David Lachapelle, 2005
Film documentary on the hip-hop dance scene in the US, by a fashion photographer.

The Rocky Horror Show
Jim Sharman, 1975
Cult film with outrageous costumes.

Saturday Night Fever
John Bradman, 1977
The disco movement explodes.

Seven Year Itch
Billy Wilder, 1955
With Marilyn Monroe and the famous scene where her dress blows up over a New York subway grill.

Shadows
John Cassavetes, 1959
New York jazz musicians in the 1950s and 1960s.

Shaft
Gordon Parks, 1971
Cult film about blaxploitation (exploitation of the black population).

Shampoo
Hal Ashby, 1975
The American jet set of the 1970s with Warren Beatty

A Streetcar named Desire
Elia Kazan, 1951
Cult film with the sleeveless tee-shirt worn by Marlon Brando.

Suzhou he
Lou Ye, 2000
Shanghai in the year 2000.

Taxi Driver
Martin Scorsese, 1976
Cult film with Robert de Niro and Jodie Foster playing a young prostitute.

The Thomas Crown Affair
Norman Jewison, 1969
Cult film about an art robbery ... with Faye Dunaway.

Traffic
Jacques Tati. 1971
Modernism as seen by Jacques Tati.

Unzipped
Douglas Keeve, 1995
Documentary on Isaac Mizrahi.

Virgin Suicides
Sofia Coppola, 1999
1970s teenage fashion in the US.

Who are you Polly Magoo?
William Klein, 1969
Fashion parody with a fashion show by Paco Rabanne.

The Wild One
Laslo Benedek, 1953
Cult film with Marlon Brando in motorbike gear.

Wild Style
Charlie Ahearn, 1982
Cult film about the beginnings of hip-hop.

The Women
George Cukor, 1939
Ten minute fashion parade included in this film about Hollywood women.

The Young Girls of Rochefort
Jacques Demy, 1967
Catherine Deneuve and Françoise Dorléac with original costumes by Jacqueline Moreau

ACKNOWLEDGEMENTS

I would like to thank:

The team at school c-6-12:
Steve Régis, assistant editor, for his research and collaboration on the organisation of the texts, Benoît Bonté for his advice on visuals, Victoria Cahouet for coordinating the visuals, Tomoe Kamiya for the fabric boards and advice on garment techniques, Martine Adrien and Jean-Philippe Bouyer for their re-reading and professional information and Masaya Ito for his active contribution.

The students for their contribution:
Angouma Poulcherie, Miwa Nakata, Ninjin Puntsag, Morgan Cahouet, Sono Fukunishi, Toshihiko Yoshino, Lei Matsuno, Li Ge, Li Chen, Jun Zhan, Juan He, Nadia Kahil, Hanako Chiba, Rumi Kikuchi, Steven Hamon, Shuntao Chen.

External contributors:
Lucie Laroche and Shunsuke Nakamura for their advice on the graphics, Antoine Kruk for his general contribution, Stephan Schopferer for his photo documentaries and general contribution to the book, Beata for her make-up, David Courtin for the image editing, Rebecca Monsarrat, Michelle...., Danaé Monseigny, Frédéric....

Fashion Professionals:
Didier Ludot for his support, preface and contribution to the vintage clothing and 'little black dress' texts.
Odile Gilbert her interview.
Stéphane Marais for his interview.
Rebecca Leach for her information on fashion photography.
Lutz Huelle for opening the doors of his studio to us and giving us an insight to his working methods.
David Ballu, financial director of the brand Lutz, for his information on how to organise a fashion company.
Le Bon Marché and Promostyl for the loan of materials.
Loulou de la Falaise

And, in particular Anne Le Bras, for the interest she has shown in my work, for her collaboration, advice, and availability throughout this project and also, for this book, which she instigated.

CREDITS

Illustrations

pp. 16, 17, 18 (left) Miwa Nakata and p.18 (right) Kana Matsunami (flower)

p. 19: Morgan Cahout

p. 20: (left) Antoine Kruk and pp. 20 and 21 (centre): Miwa Nakata

p. 30: Antoine Kruk

p. 31 Victoria Cahouet

pp. 32, 33, 34, 35: Morgan and Victoria Cahouet

pp. 36, 37: Li GE

pp. 38-53: Tomoe Kamiya and Benoit Bonte with:

Toshihiko Yoshino,

Le Ge,

Lei Chen,

Juan He and

David Courtin.

p. 40 (left), 41 (left and bottom right)

p. 42 (left), 46, (left), 47 (right) 49 (right)

p. 50 (left): Jun Zhan (illustrations)

pp. 56, 57, 58, 59: Lutz (Notebooks)

p. 63: Antoine Kruk

p. 65: Rei Matsuno

pp. 67-73: Antoine Kruk

p. 74, 75 (right): Sono Fukunishi (textile design)

p.75 (left): Antoine Kruk (illustration)

p. 77: Rei Matsuno

p.78 Jun Zhan (illustration) and Rei Matsuno (flower illustration)

pp. 90, 91: Li Zhen

pp. 96-99, 101, 104, 106, 108, 109-11: Jun Zhan

pp.118, 119 Promostyl (trend book)

pp. 120, 121, 122, 123: Hanako Chiba

p.125: Ninjin Puntsag

p. 126: Takashi Nakao

p.127: Rumi Kikuchi (tee-shirt portfolio)

p.130: Aki Shinada (portfolio)

p.131: Takashi Nakao (portfolio)

p.132 (portfolios): Takashi Nakao (top) and Hanako Chiba (bottom)

p.133 (portfolios): Takashi Nakao (top) and Rumi Kikuchi (bottom)

p.134: Nadia Kahil (portfolio)

p.135: Takashi Nakao (portfolio)

pp. 136, 137: Tomoe Kamiya (drawings, board)

p.142 (left): Lutz (research sketchbook)

p.176: Antoine Kruk (left and centre) and Benoit Bonte (right)

p. 177: Antoine Kruk

Photos

Cover : Stephan Shopferer

pp. 22, 23, 24, 25, 26, 27: Stephan Shopferer

pp. 28, 29: Stephan Shopferer (model: Victoria C, dresses by Lutz)

pp. 62, 64, 79: Shun Tao Chen (flower)

pp. 140, 141, 142 (right), 143, 144, 145, 147: Steven Shopferer

p. 150: Ninjin Punstag

pp. 156-64: Stephan Shopferer

pp. 174, 175: Olivier Gerval

pp. 178-80: Stephan Shopferer

p.181: Olivier Gerval (top) and Jules Hermant (bottom)

p. 182: David Ballu

p.183: Olivier Gerval (top) and Stephan Shopferer (bottom)

p. 184: Olivier Gerval

p.185: Olivier Gerval (top) and Stephan Shopferer (bottom)

p. 186: Olivier Gerval

p.187: Olivier Gerval (top and middle) and David Ballu (bottom)

p. 188: Olivier Gerval

p. 189: Pascal Therme

Fabrics

p.67 (skirt):	Teseo s.r.l. (T)
	Hellenic Fabrics/s.a. (H)
	Teseo s.r.l. (T)
p.68 (dress):	Komatsu Seiren (K)
	Teseo s.r.l. (T)
p.69 (trousers):	OBO (C) (Chugai Kunishima Corporation)
	Hellenic Fabrics/s.a. (H)
	Komatsu Seiren (K)
p.70 (jacket):	Nikke (N)
	Daiwabo Co. Ltd. (D)
p.71 (coat):	Leathertex (L)
	OBO (C) (Chugai Kunishima Corporation)
	Daiwabo Co. Ltd. (D)
p.72 (tee-shirt):	Nikke (N)
	Girl's (A)
p.73 (shirt):	Komatsu Seiren (K)
	Teseo s.r.l. (T)
	OBO (C) (Chugai Kunishima Corporation)
p.76 (colour variations):	Teseo s.r.l. (T)